JORDAN RUBIN

D0129269

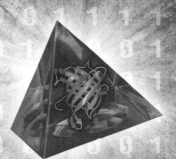

THE
VITΔMIN
CODE™

THE BREAKTHROUGH DISCOVERY THAT WILL CHANGE
THE WAY YOU TAKE VITAMINS FOREVER

MASSOUD ARVANAGHI, PHD
AND MIKE YORKEY

THE VITAMIN CODE™

The Vitamin Code

by Massoud Arvanaghi, Ph.D. and Mike Yorkey

Copyright © 2008 Garden of Life, Inc.

Brought to you by Garden of Life®, the creators of
The Vitamin Code™.

First Edition
Cover design by Dave Johnson
Interior book design by Angela Wilkeson

Garden of Life, Inc.
5500 Village Blvd.
West Palm Beach, FL 33407
(561) 748-2477

Printed in the United States of America

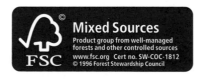

Mixed Sources
Product group from well-managed
forests and other controlled sources
www.fsc.org Cert no. SW-COC-1812
© 1996 Forest Stewardship Council
FSC

We Buy
Certified Renewable Energy
Green-e org

Our company purchases Green-
e certified renewable energy for
all of the electricity needs for
our company headquarters and
distribution center.

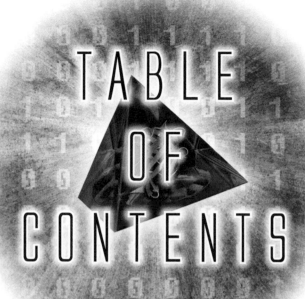

TABLE OF CONTENTS

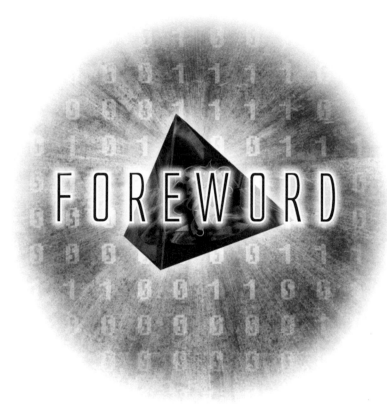

FOREWORD

BY JORDAN RUBIN

THE VITAMIN CODE™

Before my wife, Nicki, and I became the parents of three children four years of age and under, we liked to travel. Europe was always a draw for us and especially for me because of my family background. My Grandmother Rose, born in 1922 in a pastoral Polish village that could have doubled as the set for *Fiddler on the Roof,* was among the last wave of European Jews to arrive in America prior to World War II.

During the summer of 2002, Nicki and I traveled to Europe with some friends and hit all the big sights in Paris and the South of France. A side trip to picturesque Switzerland was spectacular. We stayed in the chalet-strewn village of Kandersteg, loomed over by the massive bulk of the Doldenhorn mountain. We loved the gingerbread setting and postcard Alpine vistas and hoped to return as quickly as possible.

Three years later, Nicki and I flew to Zurich for a weeklong trip to the Alps, telling ourselves that this would be a great way to celebrate our sixth wedding anniversary on September 5, 2005. There was one place I was greatly interested in visiting: the Lötschental Valley, a remote, box-canyon valley that lay on the other side of the Doldenhorn from Kandersteg. I was familiar with the Lötschental Valley from the writings of one of my health heroes, Weston A. Price, a Cleveland dentist who lived from 1870 to 1948. As he filled more and more cavities of patients sitting in his dental chair, he wondered, "Could it be our processed foods causing this dental decay?" Dr. Price left his practice and traveled around the world in the 1930s to study indigenous people whose teeth and gums were untouched by commercially made foods.

One of his stops was the Lötschental Valley, which, in the early 1930s, was virtually isolated from the rest of Switzerland. Over a two-year period, Dr. Price lived among the simple farmers and shepherds who dwelled in centuries-old wooden chalets and studied what they ate. The unaffected townsfolk, who numbered around 2,000, were surrounded on three sides by glaciers and towering granite peaks. They subsisted on what could be grown on the small plots of level land or what they raised from cows and goats grazing on lush alpine slopes in the summertime. This meant raw fruits and vegetables from their backyard plots, raw dairy products from their pasture-fed livestock, eggs from free-range chickens, and *roggenbrot*—or rye bread—from rye grown in the valley. Eating meat was a Sunday-only experience, except when bones and leftover cuts were used to make a hearty soup.

Mike and Nicole Yorkey, who had flown in from their San Diego home a few days earlier, picked us up at Zurich's Kloten Airport. Mike helps me with the research and editing for my books, and Nicole grew up in Switzerland before meeting Mike in California.

Our day trip to the Lötschental Valley—in southern Switzerland and not far from the Matterhorn—is forever etched in my mind.

First of all, modern transportation makes all the difference. We drove into the Lötschental Valley through a formidable tunnel and stopped at the first town, Wiler, where we took a cable car halfway up the Hockenhorn mountain. On this Indian Summer-like day in early September, the views of the narrow emerald-green valley lined by jutting Alpine peaks were tremendous. What lay ahead was a two-and-a-half hour hike to Fafleralp, where we could take a postal bus back to our car in Wiler. We forgot to bring along any water or food—blame it on jet lag— but fortunately there was a cute mountain restaurant along the way. We drank oversized glasses of glacier-fed water and feasted on delicious heidel berries and cream.

Fortified, we finished our scenic trek and boarded the bus for a twenty-minute ride back down the valley. Nicole, through the assistance of the local tourist office, had arranged for us to meet Ignaz Bellwald, a local historian who was born and raised in the Lötschental Valley. Unfortunately, Ignaz was born in 1940 so he had never heard of Dr. Price or his research, but he was quite content to chat away in his Swiss-German dialect while Nicole translated. He regaled us with stories, like the time when he was a young boy and chipped a tooth in half while chopping wood. Since there was no dentist in town, his uncle pulled the rest of the tooth out.

Too bad Weston A. Price wasn't around to yank Ignaz's busted tooth, but the people of the Lötschental Valley "have neither a physician nor a dentist because they have so little need for them," he wrote in his book, *Nutrition and Physical Degeneration*, which described his observations as well as his conclusions about how eating lousy foods were responsible for many of life's ills. The American dentist noted that the Lötschental adults and children had strong dispositions and sturdy bodies. Dental examinations revealed one cavity in every three mouths, or 1 percent tooth decay. Tuberculosis, which was a huge killer in the first half of the 20th century, was nonexistent in the valley. The hardy families in Lötschental Valley were incredibly healthy, and the robustness of the Lötschental men is why the Vatican pressed their young men into service as part of the Pope's Swiss Guard.

In other parts of Switzerland, though, the picture wasn't as rosy, even in the 1930s. In the major cities like Zurich and Geneva, Swiss families had access to the "diet of commerce," as Dr. Price called it, with its reliance on white flour, white sugar, and vegetable oils. They had dental cavities in one out of every three teeth, or 33 percent. Tuberculosis was a significant threat to public health. Their narrow faces contrasted with the broad, well-developed faces and palates belonging to those living in the Lötschental Valley.

The healthiness of the Lötschental people was driven home personally to me when Ignaz escorted us to Wiler's white-steeple Catholic Church. As I walked around this centuries-old house of worship, we came upon a small cemetery that drew our attention. I began reading the names and dates marking their births and deaths on the marble headstones, and I was amazed to see firsthand evidence of their long, fruitful lives. I noted the following inscriptions:

△	**Monika Tannast**	**(1898-1985)**
△	**Oliva Murmann**	**(1893-1984)**
△	**Amanda Weider**	**(1894-1982)**
△	**Theofil Murmann**	**(1903-1985)**
△	**Annamaria Kitter**	**(1891-1980)**
△	**Alina Jaggi**	**(1910-2002)**
△	**Constantina Jaggi**	**(1908-2000)**
△	**Maria Jaggi**	**(1908-2000)**
△	**Josef Seeberger**	**(1914-2000)**
△	**Katharina Ritler**	**(1894-1986)**
△	**Johann Rieder**	**(1905-1995)**
△	**Josef Murmann**	**(1889-1977)**
△	**Elizabeth Rider**	**(1908-1992)**

I'd say that 90 percent of the headstones, including the one for Ignaz's father— Viktor Bellwald (1906-1998)—showed that this cohort, mostly born at the turn of the 20th century, lived to their late eighties and early nineties. This was *fifty years longer* than the life expectancy for those born around 1900. I attributed their longevity to their diets: fresh-from-the-field raw fruits and vegetables and their grass-fed cows, sheep and goats providing high-quality dairy, and meat rich in vitamins and minerals. No "convenience foods" could be found in their wooden pantries. Their superior health and lack of dental deformities, I believe, came from consuming foods with more vitamins than found in today's foods.

I left the Lötschental Valley that day surer than ever that the typical American diet, with its heavy reliance on fast food and microwaved meals, was sending us down the road to perdition. Clearly a man ahead of his time, Dr. Price believed that restoring nutrient-dense foods into our meal plans would do us a world of good.

I'm not so sure, though, that anyone eating an all-Lötschental diet today—I'm talking about organic dairy, grass-fed beef, and several slices of roggenbrot—would receive the same bang for their nutritional buck as those mountain people did in the 1930s.

What I mean is that nearly all the foods sold in a commercial setting today, especially in our country, lack the nutritional value that our fruits, vegetables, and grains had back in the 1930s. Today's crops are grown in tired soils that have lost much of their nutrient potency over the last eight decades because of rampant mineral depletion. Since 1927, British researchers at Kings College University in London have been analyzing meat, seafood, vegetables, fruits, cereals, sugars, preserves, sweetmeats, condiments, and dairy foods as well as portions of traditional English recipes for cakes, pastries, and puddings for their organic and mineral content. We'll cut to the chase of the thirty-one page report: "The results demonstrate that there has been a significant loss of minerals and trace elements in these foods over a period of time," said the Medical Research Council.

Farmers do not allow their land to lie fallow because of the financial pressure to pay for their machinery and their debts, resorting to application of fertilizers to push up crop yields. Just look at how the economics of farming has changed farming even in the Lötschental Valley! According to Swiss records, the Lötschental Valley had two hundred farms with more than seven hundred full-time workers in the early 1930s, but by 2000, the number of farms had dropped to seventy-five and the number of full-time workers to just thirteen. It's clear that mom-and-pop farms—on both sides of the

Atlantic—can no longer compete against global agribusiness and its emphasis on large-scale farming year-after-year, season-after-season.

While modern farming techniques have achieved remarkable progress in food productivity, the downside is that fruits, vegetables, and other crops coming from our fields don't contain as many vitamins, minerals, enzymes, and beneficial microorganisms as they did in generations past. That's why I'm convinced more than ever that nutritional supplements can bridge the gap.

TURNING A PAGE

In the mid-1990s, I was struck by an illness that made me extremely nutrient deficient. I was seen by seventy doctors and medical practitioners (ranging from traditional to alternative), read more than three hundred books on health, and tried every dietary plan under the sun, from macrobiotics to metabolic typing, but none of them worked. The outlook was grim, and I was barely twenty-one years old.

It wasn't until I began following dietary principles that dated back to biblical times and trying nutritional supplements produced by probiotic fermentation that I turned a corner. The supplements contained nutrients created by beneficial microorganisms, or

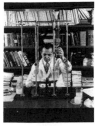

Andy Szalay in 1958

probiotics, which balanced my digestive system and enabled me to absorb the nutrients that my body needed.

I resumed a normal life. Intrigued by my progress, I began studying different compounds such as organic acids, antioxidants, and other key nutrients in an effort to formulate my own whole food nutritional supplements. In 1998 I founded a company known today as Garden of Life to introduce these nutritional supplements—similar to what I took to regain my health—to the world. The mission of Garden of Life has succeeded beyond my wildest dreams. These days, I have a solid team behind me with a mandate to create the highest-quality whole food nutritional supplements available.

Recently, an extraordinary event occurred. I was introduced to a scientist who had discovered a way to produce nutrients, vitamins, and minerals that emulated the composition of natural food. He was a Hungarian immigrant named Endre "Andy" Szalay, who founded the Grow Company, Inc., and apparently Mr. Szalay had cracked the "vitamin code" after decades of painstaking and extensive trial-and-error research. His discovery, which was so novel that the U.S. Patent Office awarded him a patent for its proprietary manufacturing technology, led to discussions about how Garden of Life and Grow Company could work together to introduce the world's first multivitamins made from raw food-created nutrients.

You'll learn more about this development later in *The Vitamin Code*, but if you're among the millions of Americans who take commercial vitamins and minerals on a regular basis, it's highly doubtful that you understand what happens when food—or any nutrient—is consumed. That is not a statement of criticism because one needs years, if not decades, of scientific study to understand how food is broken down by the body, how it's absorbed into the bloodstream, how it's delivered to the cells, and how it's utilized inside the body.

When you read *The Vitamin Code*, you'll become much more knowledgeable about the vitamins and minerals you consume.

You'll also learn more about Andy Szalay's discovery of a special process that infuses nutrients into a single-cell yeast called *Saccharomyces cerevisiae* to create vitamins and minerals that aren't isolated or synthesized, but are provided within a whole food matrix as nature intended—a discovery that was pure genius.

But quite possibly the most exciting revelation you'll find in the following pages is that by consuming Raw Food-Created Nutrients contained in The Vitamin Code™ nutritional supplements, you'll be getting these vitamins and minerals in a raw form. For the first time, individuals looking for an ideal source of essential nutrients can consume them uncooked, untreated, unadulterated, and teeming with live enzymes and probiotics to give you the most viable nutrients available today in a form the body prefers and nature provides.

We are quite fortunate to be the beneficiaries of Andy's outside-the-box thinking, especially in light of the incredibly inspirational story about how this courageous man and his family escaped to the West from behind the Iron Curtain during the Hungarian Revolution in 1956. Once you read his story in Part II, you'll have a deeper appreciation for Andy's tenacity that unlocked the Vitamin Code.

YOU'RE IN GOOD HANDS

Providing the play-by-play for *The Vitamin Code* are a pair of authors: Massoud Arvanaghi, Ph.D., and Mike Yorkey, whom I introduced earlier. Massoud—pronounced just as it looks: *Mah-sood* is a friendly, gregarious, and highly intelligent scientist who left Iran nearly thirty years ago to earn his Ph.D. studying Physical Organic Chemistry at the University of Southern California. He also received postdoctoral training in the study of advanced molecular science applications utilizing extreme environmental conditions at USC under the tutelage of George A. Olah, who would later receive a Nobel Prize for Chemistry in 1994.

Massoud—everyone calls him by his first name even though he's well earned the "Dr." salutation—has also been the co-author of more than thirty scientific articles, reviews, and patents published in major peer-reviewed American and European journals. He not only understands the science behind *The Vitamin Code*, but Massoud also has a knack for relating this complicated information in a clear, simple, and concise manner. More importantly, Massoud has worked alongside Andy Szalay at Grow Company since 1990, when he was hired to spearhead their research and product development. Massoud will be explaining what Andy's discoveries mean for us.

Joining Massoud is Mike Yorkey, who's been my researcher and editor on seventeen books, including my latest, *Perfect Weight America*. The joke is that the more we write together, the more I think we're beginning to share the same brain. His job—a tricky task—is to build the case for raw food-created nutrients while presenting the science behind *The Vitamin Code* in plain English.

I'm confident in the coming pages, *The Vitamin Code* will give you:

A greater understanding about what vitamins and minerals do in the body

An argument for Raw Food-Created Nutrients™ as the gold standard for supplementation

Insight into why most commercial vitamins are a waste of your money

By the time you finish reading *The Vitamin Code*, you'll never look at a bottle of vitamins the same again. Simply put, I believe the information contained in this book will change the way you take vitamins and minerals forever.

PART 1

A LEARNING CURVE

THE VIT∆MIN CODE™

Dawn Saunders, a San Diego mother of two preteens, doesn't shop for nutritional supplements very often. When she ventures into the vitamin aisles at a warehouse superstore or a supermarket, Dawn feels like she's stepping into alien territory, a place where she's ill-equipped to determine what vitamins and minerals are best to purchase for her family and herself. From her point of view, too many manufacturers offer too many choices on too many store shelves. She feels that she somehow lacks the information and the nutritional expertise to make wise choices.

So Dawn keeps things simple and sticks to what she knows. These days, calcium and chewable vitamin C are the only bottles of nutritional supplements that earn a place in her shopping cart—as long as they're on sale. "Supplements are expensive," she said, "so I choose my vitamins wisely. Calcium is important to me because the kids don't drink milk. I can get them to take chewable vitamin C as long as they're sweet-tasting."

She and her husband, Rick, are the parents of twelve-year-old Sydney and ten-year-old Cole, and like every mother and father, they want their children—on the cusp of adolescence—to grow up strong and healthy. "My overall philosophy is that if we eat from all the food groups, then everyone should be getting their nutritional needs met," she said. "But the kids are not big veggie eaters. They are picky about what they like to eat, so I wonder what I should do to fill in the gap."

Millions of parents as well as consumers wonder what steps they should take to fill in the nutritional potholes in their diets. They are concerned, and rightly so, that their bodies are not receiving all the vitamins and minerals they need, whether it's from a distaste for green salads and fiber-rich vegetables or their preference for "comfort" foods high in taste, high in calories—and low in nutritive value. They've also heard that today's fresh fruits and vegetables, as well as our frozen and commercially prepared foods, don't pack the same nutritional zip as they did for our forefathers, but they're not sure how to act upon that information. Bottom line: they fear that their erratic eating habits, punctuated with a heavy reliance on fast-food meals on-the-go, home-delivered pizza, and sugary desserts don't ensure an adequate supply of essential nutrients and beneficial compounds necessary for optimal health.

Maybe you see yourself in Dawn Saunders' flip-flops, conscious that nutritional supplements could compensate for any dietary inadequacies in your family, but feeling overwhelmed by the hundreds of choices on health food or grocery store shelves. If so, you're not alone. The task of educating yourself about vitamins and minerals can be challenging at best and daunting at worst.

This book, *The Vitamin Code*, will attempt to bridge that gap. In the following pages, we'll not only make the case for why you and your family should take nutritional supplements, but we'll explain why a class of vitamins and minerals made from raw food-created nutrients raises the bar on nutritional supplementation.

You see, not all vitamin and mineral supplements are the same. They vary widely in their source material and the manufacturing methods used to create them. They vary widely in their potency and effectiveness. And they vary widely in price, as Dawn Saunders has discovered. Despite these broad differences, the weak nutritional value of conventional crops, an increase in environmental pollution, and the stresses of modern living means that nutritional supplementation is more important than ever. It becomes increasingly harder and harder to obtain the minimum recommended amounts of vitamins and minerals solely from today's diet.

Taking nutritional supplementation is no longer a fad, but part of a growing trend for parents like Dawn Saunders, who seek out a proactive approach to their health and the health of their loved ones. The key is understanding what the *very best* vitamin and mineral supplements are for your situation. By the time you finish reading *The Vitamin Code*, we're confident that you'll know what path to follow as you seek out the path to extraordinary health for you and your family.

ARE SUPPLEMENTS NECESSARY?

No one wants to get ripped off, and everyone wants to be healthy. So are taking vitamin supplements an expensive way to produce urine the color of lemonade or a smart insurance policy for eating today's less-than-nutritious diet?

We do know that the Journal of the American Medical Association (JAMA) reversed its policy several years ago and now recommends that adults take at least one multivitamin a day. Some however, say that taking vitamins probably won't hurt you but quickly add that they won't help you. Others adopt a laissez-faire approach, saying, "If you're taking a multivitamin, there's no reason to stop. But if you're not taking a multivitamin, there's also no reason to start taking one, either."

Such a take-it-or-leave-it attitude belies growing evidence that our foods do not contain the vitamins, minerals, enzymes, and beneficial microorganisms that they did a hundred years ago because they are grown in nutrient-barren soils that have been doused with pesticides and herbicides. Yesterday's foods fueled Ben-Hur;

today's foods power Pee Wee Herman.

Then there's the issue of genetically modified foods. Just as few consumers are aware that they've been purchasing vitamins made from synthetic isolates, you're probably unaware that you've been eating genetically modified foods for some time. It's estimated that 75 percent of the processed foods in this country (including breakfast cereals, baked goods, and vegetable oils) contain a potpourri of genetically modified organisms. This is an amazing development since GMO crops such as corn, soybeans, and potatoes have only been around since the mid-1990s.

Called the "food of the future" by proponents and "Frankenfood" by detractors, GMO crops are created by taking genes from one organism—often a mutated virus— and inserting them into another to make them grow higher, larger, denser, and more resistant to insect infestation. Those are all laudable goals, but the problem is that scientists are adding a gene to a food that wasn't originally part of that food, which is unnatural and changes the DNA character of the crop.

Meanwhile, the quality of our food supply continues to hemorrhage. A comparison of U.S. Department of Agriculture food composition tables from the 1960s and 1970s to the present day reveals that the vitamin and mineral content of the nation's breadbasket has declined an average of 20 percent in the last generation. Another overlooked factor is the need to move fruits and vegetables long distances, which is good for the trucking industry but lousy for our nutrition since shipping produce thousands of miles doesn't allow fruits and vegetables to mature. These foods must be picked before they reach the peak of ripeness, or they'll arrive half-rotten and squishy before they're even set for sale in our nation's supermarkets.

The case for taking nutritional supplements has never been stronger.

LOOKING BACK AT HISTORY

Still not convinced? Perhaps we should take a few steps backward before we go forward. A good place to begin would be to relate some basic information on what vitamins are. The classic definition for vitamins is that they consist of a group of multifaceted organic substances that regulate metabolism and are required in our daily diets for normal growth and maintenance of life. In plain English, vitamins are extremely complex substances or micronutrients needed for the human body to work correctly.

The scientific discovery that vitamins and minerals exist is not that old—just a hundred years, as we'll soon explain. Up until a century ago, scientists and doctors of the day could only make educated guesses that there had to be *something* in foods that provided us with health and well-being. After all, even the most casual observer of the human condition understood that food was a source of energy and sustained life. Since time immemorial, sick people had relied on folk medicine or "old wives' tales" to tell them that certain foods could cure whatever ailed them.

But what was *inside* the foods? For a long time, mankind didn't have a very good idea. A classic example happened in the 15th century when sailors began dying of scurvy during tedious three-month journeys to the New World. Scurvy was a nasty disease, marked by general weakness, joint pain, bleeding of the gums, loose teeth, and blood spots appearing all over the body. Death came suddenly—in the "middle of a sentence" according to one account—when a main artery burst. Half of the unlucky crew who signed on to Portuguese navigator Vasco da Gama's long voyage around the Cape of Good Hope (1497-1499) perished from scurvy, which meant da Gama's long expedition around the southern tip of Africa couldn't have been a pleasure cruise.

Doctors and scientists back then didn't know that scurvy resulted from a lack of vitamin C in the diet. Nor were they aware that vitamin C was found in citrus fruits such as oranges, lemons, limes, and grapefruit, and also in tomatoes, potatoes, cabbage, and green peppers. Meanwhile, scurvy remained a vexing problem on the ocean blue since sailing ships didn't have refrigeration to stock perishable fruits and vegetables in their holds.

The deadly disease also struck those left behind on land. Medieval adults and children on *terra firma* succumbed when fresh fruits and vegetables weren't available during the winter months—or times of famine and plague. In the 16th and 17th centuries, more than one hundred scurvy epidemics ravaged Europe, including Ireland's Great Potato Famine. (Potatoes contain vitamin C and were the Irish's main source of that vitamin.)

Medical experts at the time thought scurvy was something contagious but had no idea what brought on the deadly disease. It wasn't until 1747 when a Scottish naval surgeon, James Lind, happened upon a dramatic cure without understanding that vitamin C was involved. During one experiment, Dr. Lind treated scurvy-ridden sailors with lemons and oranges. Overnight, they rebounded from death's door. Despite this discovery that *something* in the citrus fruits kept seafarers from contracting scurvy, it was still another 50 years before the British Navy stocked their ship holds with lime juice. (And now you know why the British are called "limeys" in period Hollywood films.)

Scurvy is a historical footnote today since supermarkets readily stock dozens of fruits and vegetables rich in vitamin C the entire year. Yet even with an abundance of farm-fresh produce available on store shelves year round, doctors today are seeing patients with significant vitamin and mineral deficiencies. Baby boomers— especially older women—lack enough vitamin D and calcium in their blood to prevent osteoporosis, a disease in which bones become brittle and threaten to break. Bone loss accelerates after menopause when estrogen levels decline; we've all seen the sad image of a woman hunched over with a dowager's hump. In a review of women with osteoporosis that were hospitalized for hip fractures, 50 percent were found to have signs of vitamin D deficiency, according to the National Institutes of Health.

Rickets, another bone-debilitating disease, has made a comeback in recent years among children. Two hundred years ago, rickets was so common in poorer parts of Dickensian England that it was called "The English Disease." Once scientists discovered in the 20th century that vitamin D eradicated rickets, the disease became so rare that the U.S. government stopped keeping statistics on it. Despite all that we know about its root causes, rickets has made a resurgence today because of a lack of vitamin D in children's diets as well as kids' propensity to stay indoors. Vitamin D is nicknamed the "sunshine vitamin" because the body manufactures it from the ultraviolet rays of the sun.

Other diseases and ailments are gaining ground these days, despite all that we know about vitamins, minerals, and good nutrition. A deficiency in riboflavin, for example, results from a diet missing meat, fish, legumes, and green leafy vegetables. Vegans, who don't eat any meat, fish, dairy products, or eggs, must guard against low intake of riboflavin, which is important in converting protein, fats, and carbohydrates into energy, as well as repairing body tissues. Vitamin B12, found primarily in meat, dairy products, and eggs is another cause for concern for vegans since it's also absent in plant foods. A vitamin B12 deficiency could lead to pernicious anemia.

The point is that despite the knowledge of modern science, the universal agreement that the body needs a wide range of vitamins and minerals, and the ability to shop year-round for healthy, nutritious foods, we are still falling short of leading healthy, vibrant lives. Our nutritional deficiencies may not cause noticeable health disorders, but they can result in a variety of symptoms along with a general decrease in wellness. Unaddressed, these nutritional deficiencies can often put the body at risk for future health problems. In a sense, you could be sailing through life, unaware that the foods you eat or the type of vitamins and minerals you take could shipwreck your health.

AN IMPORTANT SCIENTIFIC BREAKTHROUGH

As mentioned previously, none of vitamins discussed so far—vitamin C, vitamin D, vitamin B2 (riboflavin), or vitamin B12 (cyanocobalamin)—had been "discovered" a hundred years ago. In the 1800s, the baseline of scientific knowledge was that humans needed to consume the proteins in meat, the carbohydrates in grains, the fats in dairy, and a little salt to stay healthy. No one had ever heard of vitamins.

Scientific researchers in the late 1800s and early 1900s were becoming more and more aware, however, that certain factors in food were responsible for preventing disease. Christiaan Eijkman, a Dutch physician and pathologist, was dispatched to Indonesia by the Dutch East India Company in 1886 to deal with a great horror—*beriberi,* one of the most common diseases in the Far East and a Singhalese word for extreme weakness. Victims of beriberi contended with weight loss, weakness and pain in the limbs, and impaired sensory perception. They lost nearly all mobility before their hearts gave out. Autopsies showed that the nerve fibers and heart muscles had degenerated.

Dr. Eijkman joined a Dutch East India scientific team that looked at everything they could under a microscope: blood, saliva, and urine. Nothing out of the ordinary presented itself. After nine months in the Indonesian bush, the Dutch team sailed home, leaving behind their youngest member—Dr. Eijkman—to keep an eye on things. For ten *years* Dr. Eijkman kept plugging away until one day he noticed that the institute's chickens were coming down with beriberi-like symptoms: an inability to walk steadily or peck for food. Many keeled over and died. Then one day, the ailing chickens suddenly recovered.

What gave? Dr. Eijkman wasn't sure. He asked the cook what he was feeding the chickens, and he replied that he had given the chickens bowls of white rice because the usual shipment of cheaper brown rice hadn't shown up. Polished white rice was more expensive because a "refinement" process stripped away the outer husks and shined up the rice hulls to a glossy sheen. In Victorian times, Europeans thought eating polished white rice made the dining experience more civilized instead of swallowing the tougher-to-chew brown rice.

When the cook's boss found out that the chickens were eating the expensive white rice, he blew a gasket. The chickens were immediately put back on a brown rice diet—and that's when their barnyard health improved.

Dr. Eijkman struggled to figure out this conundrum. White rice: chickens sick. Brown rice: chickens well. Maybe there was poison in the white rice. Maybe there was an antidote in brown rice. Who else was eating white rice and brown rice that he could check out? The answer: prisoners. The Dutch physician checked the local jails to see what kind of rice was slopped onto prisoner's tin plates. Where convicts were served white rice, beriberi reared its ugly head. Where prisoners ate brown rice, beriberi wasn't a problem.

Dr. Eijkman's assumption was that a toxin, or poison, within the kernel of white rice was neutralized by something in the outer husk. His research was cut short, however, when illness forced Dr. Eijkman's return to the Netherlands in 1896. Upon his arrival in the Old World, he told his colleagues, "White rice can be poisonous!" —a declaration that probably stunted sales of refined white rice in the food markets of Amsterdam and The Hague.

But the Dutch researcher was on to something.

Meanwhile, back in Indonesia, a colleague named Gerrit Grijns stepped into the position held by Dr. Eijkman. In 1901, Grijns proposed that beriberi was not caused by some mysterious toxin or deadly germs but by the lack of a vital substance contained in the outer husks. He was the first to suggest that beriberi could actually be a dietary deficiency disease.

Five years later, English biochemist F. G. Hopkins advanced the idea that foods contain certain substances needed to sustain life itself. Through his feeding experiments with laboratory animals, he concluded that foods must contain necessary "accessory factors" in addition to proteins, carbohydrates, fats, salts, and water.

THESE FACTORS WERE DEFINED AS:

1. Substances found to be absolutely necessary for life to continue.

2. Substances that the body could not synthesize on its own.

The British scientist didn't know what to call these substances, however.

A Polish colleague, Casimir Funk, Ph.D., connected the dots in 1912 by isolating the active substances in rice husks that were preventing beriberi. He named this anti-beriberi factor a "vitamine"—the prefix "vita" being the Latin word for life and suffix "amine" referring to his belief that it was an amine, or compound, derived from ammonia. Further research revealed, however, that not all organic molecules contained amines, so the letter "e" was dropped in 1920 when it was clear that not all vitamins were amines.[1]

Your head may be spinning following this avalanche of information, but the upshot of this early 20th century research is that Hopkins and Funk formulated the vitamin hypothesis of deficiency disease, which is another way of saying that if you don't receive the necessary vitamins from the foods you eat, you could face a life-threatening disease or live a far from healthy skip-to-my-lou existence. They contended that "factors" in meat, dairy, fruits, and vegetables—the vitamins and minerals—played a significant nutritional role in our lives, and they believed that one day science would bear their theories out.

Ever since the discovery of these essential life substances in food, however, scientists have debated the issue of nutritional adequacy. It's a debate that still rages today among researchers who have yet to unlock the "vitamin code."

[1] Fittingly, Drs. Eijkman and Hopkins shared the 1929 Nobel Prize in Physiology and Medicine.

IN ALPHABETICAL ORDER

The pioneering work of Drs. Eijkman, Hopkins, and Funk undoubtedly advanced scientific knowledge and led to additional discoveries in the world of biochemical nutrition. By the 1930s, biochemists had discerned thirteen vitamins and divided them into two primary classes according to their solubility in water or fats. Those that dissolved in fat, or are fat-soluble, were vitamins A, D, E, and K. Those that dissolved in water, or were water-soluble, were vitamin C and a group of molecules referred to as the vitamin B complex such as vitamin B1, B2, biotin, and folic acid.

Up until 1920, scientists called these substances "fat-soluble A," "water-soluble B," and "water-soluble C" until Jack Cecil Drummond, a British biochemist, recommended that this "somewhat cumbrous nomenclature" be dropped in favor of referring to them as vitamins A, B, and C, etc.

It's important to be aware of the distinctions between the fat-soluble and water-soluble vitamins, though. Since fat-soluble vitamins can be stored in fat cells, your body keeps a supply of these vitamins available for use on demand. The downside is that toxic levels can build up in the body, leading to potentially severe side effects.

Water-soluble vitamins, on the other hand, are stored in the body in small amounts. Any quantity not put to good use right away is quickly excreted by the body, which explains why you have bright yellow, glow-in-the-dark urine within an hour of popping several tablets of vitamin B2 and/or vitamin C.

Since all vitamins are essential nutrients required for normal chemical processes to occur in the body and each vitamin plays a unique role within the body, let's look over a breakdown of different vitamin types:

THE FAT-SOLUBLE VITAMINS

Fat-soluble vitamins require the presence of fat carriers in the body to be absorbed and thus are not as easily assimilated as water-soluble vitamins. Once these vitamins are absorbed in the bloodstream from the intestinal tract, they support important functions like cell division, bone development, and eyesight. Excess fat-soluble vitamins are stored in the liver or the adipose tissue.

If your diet is tilted toward the consumption of fat-free foods, then you should know that these so-called "diet" foods interfere with fat-soluble vitamins because fatty acids are needed for their absorption. In fact, due to the large consumption of these diet foods today, many researchers believe that adequate amounts of these important fat-soluble vitamins are missing from the diets of many Americans.

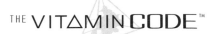

THE LIST OF FΛT-SOLUBLE VITΛMINS:

VITΛMIN Λ

Here is a vitamin essential to many bodily processes, from maintaining healthy skin to regulating the immune system. Vitamin A plays an important role in vision, bone growth, and cell division. Vitamin A deficiency is the leading cause of preventable blindness in children and increases the risk of disease and death from severe infections. A lack of vitamin A can lead to night blindness and other eye problems as well as problems in pregnancy, including a higher risk of maternal mortality.

Sources of vitamin A are foods that come from animals, such as meat, eggs, milk, and cheese. Vitamin A from plant sources like carrots, spinach, cantaloupes, apricots, and sweet potatoes is called beta carotene or pro-vitamin A, but the body can't absorb vitamin A from plant sources as well as it can from animal foods.

Heavy drinkers of alcohol deplete their stores of vitamin A. Deficiencies can also occur when vitamin A is lost through chronic diarrhea. Vitamin A was discovered in 1913 when scientists showed that butter and egg yolk contained a substance necessary for healthy growth in laboratory animals.

VITΛMIN D

Vitamin D is not actually a vitamin but a hormone that regulates the formation of our skeletal system as well as enhancing the absorption of calcium and phosphorus from the intestine. Vitamin D aids the function of the nervous system. As parents of young children like Dawn Saunders know, vitamin D is crucial for growing young bones and new teeth. Many parents aren't aware, however, that vitamin D helps the body absorb calcium, which is essential for bone growth.

Foods rich in vitamin D are fatty fish such as salmon and tuna, high omega-3 eggs, whole milk, and other dairy products, preferably raw and not homogenized and pasteurized. Remember how in the Foreword that Jordan Rubin mentioned the findings of Dr. Weston A. Price? Price also noted that the diet of the Lötschental people contained "at least ten times" the amount of fat-soluble vitamins as compared to the standard American diet. That's because raw dairy products are one of the top sources of vitamin D.

Besides targeting foods high in vitamin D, don't forget that exposure to sunlight on the skin allows the body to manufacture this vital vitamin from the sun's ultraviolet light. Living north of an east-west line connecting Philadelphia and San Francisco, however, increases the odds for not getting enough vitamin D, especially in northern regions of the country noted for their cold, gray winters. Sorry about that, Buffalo, but the low angle of the winter sun doesn't provide enough ultraviolet light.

VITAMIN E

Here's another crucial fat-soluble vitamin that supports the body with the formation of red blood cells. Vitamin E is a potent antioxidant that has a powerfully positive effect. This essential vitamin also protects your cells against the effects of free radicals, which are oxygen molecules with a single electron hell-bent on attacking cell life in your body and may contribute to the development of disease. Sources of vitamin E are whole grains, corn, green leafy vegetables, spinach, broccoli, asparagus, almonds, peanut butter, sunflower seeds, olives, egg yolks, and fruits like kiwi and mangos. Organ meats, seafood, and wheat germ oil are also top sources.

VITΛMIN K

You don't hear much about vitamin K, but in case you're wondering, this unique vitamin has nothing to do with a certain breakfast cereal. What Vitamin K does is help the body maintain normal levels of blood-clotting proteins, prevent oxidative cell damage, and aid in the maintenance of bone mass.

The good news is that most adults have no problem receiving enough vitamin K. In addition, it's rare to have a true deficiency of vitamin K because our intestinal bacteria readily manufacture it. Promising vitamin K research shows that even though deficiencies of vitamin K are rare, consuming both known forms of vitamin K, K1 and K2, can derive excellent health benefits. Sources of vitamin K are similar to vitamin E: leafy green vegetables, egg yolks, and dairy products. Green foods—alfalfa, wheatgrass, and barley grass—also contain generous amounts of vitamin K.

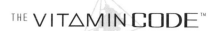
WATER-SOLUBLE VITAMINS

Water-soluble vitamins are not stored in the body and thus need regular replenishment. Since these vitamins dissolve in water, the body can quickly eliminate excess or unused amounts through urination. Water-soluble vitamins are easily destroyed or washed out during food storage and preparation, so it's important to consume fresh fruits and vegetables, keep milk and grains away from strong light, and use the cooking water from vegetables to prepare soups.

VITAMIN B-COMPLEX

The B vitamins are known to be an eight-member family, although scientists will argue there are more likely twenty or more B vitamins in existence. The eight B vitamins are thiamine (B1), riboflavin (B2), niacin (nicotinic acid), pyridoxine (B6), folic acid, cyanocobalamin (B12), biotin (vitamin H), and pantothenic acid (B3).

B vitamins generate energy that the body taps into to carry out its activities. They are responsible for making red blood cells that carry oxygen to various parts of the body. Rich sources of B vitamins include whole grains such as wheat and oats, brewer's and baker's yeast, fish and seafood, leafy green vegetables, dairy products including milk and yogurt, and legumes like beans and peas.

Λ QUICK SNΛPSHOT OF EΛCH OF THE EIGHT B VITΛMINS:

- **Thiamine or B1** helps release energy from food, promotes a normal appetite, and supports normal nerve and heart function. It's also been called a "morale vitamin" because of its importance to maintaining a good mood. Sources are whole grains, rice husk, yeast, liver, eggs, milk, green leaves, and meat.

- **Riboflavin or Vitamin B2** is responsible for body growth and red blood cell production, helps in releasing energy from carbohydrates, and keeps mucous membranes healthy. Sources are whole grains, malted barley, dark green vegetables, eggs, milk, kidney, heart, and liver.

- **Niacin** works closely with vitamins B1, B2, B6, pantothenic acid, and biotin to break the carbohydrates, fats, and proteins in food down into energy. Good sources of niacin include liver, yeast, poultry, fish, alfalfa, corn, and legumes like peas and beans.

- **Vitamin B6** aids in red blood cell formation and helps the body use fats. Sources are yeast, whole grains, liver, and green leafy vegetables.

- **Folic Acid** provides normal growth and maintenance of all cells and produces neurotransmitters such as serotonin, which regulates mood, sleep, and appetite. Good sources of folic acid are mushrooms, yeast, peas, wheat germ, peanuts, spinach, dark green vegetables, and organ meats.

- **Biotin** helps the body use protein, fat, and carbohydrates for energy. Good sources of biotin are meats and liver, egg yolks, milk, peanuts, yeast, and whole grains.

- **Pantothenic Acid** is essential to the metabolism of carbohydrates, proteins, and fats, as well as for the synthesis of hormones and cholesterol. Good sources are liver, rice bran, molasses, meat, poultry, fish, dairy products, whole grains, broccoli, cauliflower, and legumes.

VITAMIN C

Vitamin C, probably the best-known vitamin in your pantry or kitchen cabinet, strengthens gums and teeth, and forms collagen as a basis for healthy bones, muscles, and skin. In addition, the body calls upon vitamin C to maintain the health and proper function of the immune system. Vitamin C, as mentioned earlier, is found in citrus fruits, rose hips, strawberries, acerola cherries, fresh tea leaves, green and red peppers, tomatoes, broccoli, spinach, and cabbage.

DON'T FORGET THE MINERALS

Similar to vitamins, minerals enable the body to perform many functions, including energy production, growth, and healing. You need minerals because they act as catalysts for many biological reactions within the body, including muscle response, the transmission of messages through the nervous system, the production of hormones, digestion, and the utilization of nutrients in foods. All tissues and internal bodily fluids contain varying quantities of minerals, and minerals are components of bones, teeth, soft tissue, muscle, blood, and nerve cells. While the body can manufacture some vitamins, such as vitamin D, the body cannot manufacture a single mineral.

The Big Seven—calcium, chloride, magnesium, phosphorous, potassium, sodium and sulfur—are minerals needed only in small amounts, but their absence is keenly felt by the body, resulting in poor health and sometimes death. In addition, the number of trace minerals essential to life now exceeds thirty.

NUTRITION IN A BOTTLE

As scientific knowledge about nutrition grew by leaps and bounds in the 1920s and 1930s, rapid changes in the manufacture and production of food were happening as well. The Industrial Revolution gave mankind the technology to change from an agrarian society to a modern industrial society relying on complex machinery. Methods of food preparation also experienced dramatic changes. Canning factories and commercial bakeries sprouted up like spring flowers, producing attractive and marketable food products that could be shipped long distances. Instead of preparing foods from scratch at home—picking veggies from the backyard garden, plucking chickens, churning butter, milling flour—Americans could walk into a neighborhood market and purchase canned fruits and vegetables, boxes of cereal, and packaged cookies and cakes.

And now you know why dentists like Weston A. Price could afford to take a two-year sabbatical from filling cavities.

Health-minded individuals back in the 1930s had already figured out that processed foods were detrimental to good health. They were the first to promulgate the idea that we should supplement our diets because the newfangled foods of the "modern diet" were produced from storehouses of refined white flour, processed refined oils, and refined sugar. During the Great Depression, we started to see the first dietary supplements on the market, which were actually a mixture of wheat and barley grass that could be mixed into your favorite juice or milk. These cereal grasses, as they were known, became very popular.

Flash forward seventy-five years to today, where the prevailing conventional wisdom states that consuming vitamins and minerals is a good idea—kind of like flossing. Most likely, since you're holding this book, you and your family agree, and you take some sort of nutritional supplements on a regular basis. You're not alone: It's estimated that 68 percent of American adults avail themselves of at least one commercial nutritional supplement, according to a recent survey conducted for the Council for Responsible Nutrition, a Washington, D.C.-based trade association representing ingredient suppliers and manufacturers in the dietary supplement industry. The survey also revealed that 52 percent of adults consider themselves to be regular users of nutritional supplements. With the number of American adults age 18 and over numbering around 225 million, this effectively means that more than 117 million adults regularly take nutritional supplements.[2]

Sales of supplements totaled $22 billion in 2007, according to *Nutrition Business Journal* statistics. That works out to $60 million spent *per day* at the checkout register. Within these sales, the top eight nutritional supplements purchased were (in descending order):

1. **Multivitamins**
2. **Calcium**
3. **Vitamin C**
4. **Fish Oil**
5. **Vitamin E**
6. **Antioxidants**
7. **Vitamin B/B Complex**
8. **Omega-3s**

[2] The Vitamin Code will not be discussing the nutritional supplement needs of children, nor should the recommendations in this book be applied to children under the age of six.

With such a large financial opportunity, thousands of companies covet their slice of the pie and compete for your hard-earned dollars through clever marketing, brilliant packaging, or superior pricing. In the war to reach the consumer, however, the first casualty is often the truth—as well as candor. No advertising campaigns trumpet the fact that their vitamins and minerals are produced from synthetic source materials that merely *imitate* the original nutrients found in food.

What happened is that back in the 1930s and 1940s, biochemists were having success isolating the active "factors" that F.G. Hopkins first hypothesized about back in 1906. These scientists discovered that the thirteen vitamins were made up of a complex set of interrelated compounds that they called "co-factors." They included:

△ Precursers   △ Enzymes

△ Co-Enzymes   △ Trace-Element Activators

△ Amino Acids   △ Bioflavonoids

△ Co-Vitamins   △ Co-Minerals

△ Essential Fatty Acids   △ Phytonutrients

△ Micronutrients

Once chemists were able to separate or characterize this molecular information—a process called isolation—they were able to reproduce the vitamin's molecular structure in the lab by using specific chemical reactions. In other words, biochemists in their white lab coats peered through their microscopes and figured out ways to synthetically create (or imitate) complex structures such as vitamin E, vitamin C, and beta-carotene. While these isolated nutrients are representative of man's genius inside the laboratory, they were also nutritional folly because they skipped the entire process of nature—and removed, decreased or simply left out some of the vital "co-factors" that occur naturally in food.

Let's use beta-carotene, which the body converts into vitamin A, as an example. When beta-carotene was isolated in the laboratory, the lab scientists couldn't include important co-factors such as alpha, beta, gamma, and delta carotenes; lycopene; lutein; zeaxanthin; cryptoxanthin; phytoene, phytofluene, and neurosporene. That's not even a complete list, but that hasn't stopped vitamin companies from selling you bottles marked with "Beta-Carotene" on the label.

Whenever you pop a couple of synthetically produced capsules of beta-carotene down the hatch, the body attempts to "build" a complete vitamin complex by adding the missing co-factors that it knows should be there. The AWOL co-factors must be replaced from either the foods you eat or from the body's stores.

We would venture that 99 percent of the 117 million Americans who regularly take nutritional supplements have no idea that they've been sold a pig in a poke. When I (Mike Yorkey) escorted Dawn Saunders through several aisles of nutritional supplements at a San Diego health food store, she was blissfully unaware that the active ingredient for vitamin C, a supplement she regularly shops for, was made up of a synthetically produced nutrient: ascorbic acid. Furthermore, she believed any price differential was based on the number of tablets inside the plastic bottle or some other feature, like whether the vitamin C was chewable or not.

Dawn represents the vast majority of shoppers for nutritional supplements, pursuing certain vitamins and minerals for the benefit they could bring her family but unaware of their composition or quality. If you're among this group, please pay attention to the following story, which is essential to understanding the need for the information contained in this book, *The Vitamin Code*.

HOW VITΛMIN C CΛME TO BE

Our story begins in Hungary at the turn of the 20th century. Albert Szent-Györgyi (pronounced Sent-Jor-jyee), born in 1893 to a prominent Budapest family, started university studies at the age of eighteen at the Budapest Medical School. Bored with his pre-med classes but inquisitive about science, he enjoyed hanging out at his uncle's anatomy lab at the University of Budapest and looking over some shoulders. Uncle Mihály Lenhossék allowed him to stay on one condition, however: that his first research project would zero in on the human rectum and anus. (His poor uncle, who suffered from painful hemorrhoids, hoped to profit from his nephew's . . . ah . . . explorations.)

Szent-Györgyi didn't shrink from the challenge. He dove wholeheartedly into the task at hand, and his first scientific article, published in 1913 at the age of twenty, dealt with the epithelium of the anus, or the tissues of the anal cavity. "Because of my uncle," he joked later, "I started science at the wrong end."

Life would take an unwelcome turn when his medical studies were interrupted by the outbreak of World War I in 1914. The Hungarian Army sent him out to the battlefield as a medic, a gruesome job in an era of bullets and bayonets. After two years of dragging shot-up comrades off the front lines, he despaired of surviving the trench warfare that chewed up so many young lives like hamburger. Disgusted with the war, he carefully and calmly fired a pistol into his upper arm, claiming he was hit by enemy fire. The ruse worked, and he was discharged from military service.

Szent-Györgyi finished his medical education, became an M.D. in 1917, and married. For the next eleven years, he conducted research at several universities, including the University of Groningen in the Netherlands, studying the chemistry of cellular respiration. His excellent work attracted the attention of Cambridge University, where he worked with F.G. Hopkins. It was in England that Szent-Györgyi became interested in the "browning" or oxidation process that occurs when a slice of apple is exposed to the air. Szent-Györgyi found out he could delay the browning with the addition of citrus juice or speed it up with the introduction of peroxidase, an enzyme active in oxidation. Further experiments allowed Szent-Györgyi to isolate the protective agent in citrus juice, which he christened "hexuronic acid."

Szent-Györgyi returned to his homeland in 1931 when he accepted a position at the University of Szeged and continued his research into hexuronic acid. His new responsibilities included teaching, and he soon established a reputation for fascinating lectures and an informal leadership style. He played sports with his students and loved to ride his bicycle across campus to visit colleagues.

One of those colleagues was an American post-doctoral fellow, Joseph Svirbely, who joined Szent-Györgyi's research team. Svirbely had been working with C.G. King at the University of Pittsburgh on trials to isolate vitamin C. Szent-Györgyi asked Svirbely to test some hexuronic acid on guinea pigs with scurvy-like symptoms. The trial indicated that foods enriched with hexuronic acid helped the guinea pigs recover, but foods without hexuronic acid exacerbated the guinea pigs' scurvy condition. Szent-Györgyi decided that hexuronic acid was the long-sought-after vitamin C.

Svirbely wrote his former mentor, C.G. King, telling him what they had discovered in their Szeged laboratory, adding that he and Szent-Györgyi were going to submit their study to *Nature*, a scientific journal. A month later, *Science* published an announcement from C.G. King that he had discovered vitamin C, which was identical to hexuronic acid. King cited Szent-Györgyi's earlier work but failed to give him any credit.

The discovery story was major news and widely disseminated by American newspapers. The news traveled fast to Europe, and when Szent-Györgyi and Svirbely heard about it, they felt they had been betrayed. They quickly sent off their own report to *Nature*, challenging King's assertion that he was the first to discover vitamin C. A bitter controversy erupted in the scientific world.

Apart from who got there first, Szent-Györgyi had a more immediate problem: he had used up all his hexuronic acid with the guinea pigs experiment. He tried extracting hexuronic acid from oranges, lemons, and limes because of their proven anti-scurvy properties, but the sugars in the citrus fruits made purification extremely difficult. Szent-Györgyi cast about for other foods that could possibly contain hexuronic acid. One night, his wife served him fresh red paprika with their dinner meal. Nothing unusual about that; Szeged prided itself as the "Paprika Capital of the World," a city where restaurants placed matching salt and paprika shakers on every table.

As he wrote in his autobiography, "I did not feel like eating it [the paprika], so I thought of a way out. Suddenly it occurred to me that this is the one plant I had never tested. I took it to the laboratory . . . [and by] about midnight I knew that it was a treasure chest full of vitamin C."

After this pivotal moment, Szent-Györgyi knew he was on to something. He immediately mobilized his staff for a large-scale extraction of hexuronic acid from Hungarian paprika. After a couple of dozen steps of isolation, purification, and crystallization, they produced a little more than a kilo of white crystalline powder. Instead of calling it hexuronic acid, Szent Györgyi renamed it "a-scorbic" acid since it prevented *scorbutus*, a formal name for scurvy.

The scientific community credited Szent-Györgyi for being the first to successfully "isolate vitamin C in the form of ascorbic acid and awarded him the Nobel Prize in 1937. News of Szent-Györgyi winning science's most prestigious award turned him into an overnight celebrity in Hungary and around the world. A *Time* magazine feature story dated November 1, 1937, said, "In his own backyard, this far-traveling researcher found that paprika was the best source of vitamin C on earth." As winner of the Nobel Prize for Medicine, Szent-Györgyi collected $40,000, worth $585,000 in today's dollars. Now he was famous *and* wealthy.

Szent-Györgyi didn't rest on his laurels, but his next discovery was totally unexpected. In this experiment, a concentrated form of ascorbic acid extracted from paprika was given to patients with purplish patches on their skin due to localized spontaneous bleeding. The patients made rapid recoveries after being treated with this ascorbic acid, or vitamin C. Next, Szent-Györgyi and his colleagues gave another set of patients with purplish patches an even purer solution of ascorbic acid, thinking that 100 percent ascorbic acid would cure patients *even* faster. Yet the opposite occurred; the pure ascorbic acid had very little effect on the patients.

"When I had crystalline ascorbic acid, we tried it again, expecting a still stronger reaction," Szent-Györgyi wrote in his memoirs. "It did nothing. Evidently, my impure extract contained an additional substance responsible for the reaction. I guessed that it might be 'flavones,' which did the trick. My guess proved right. I isolated the flavones from paprika, and they helped the patients get better. I called this group of substances 'vitamin P.' I used the letter P because I was not quite sure that it was a vitamin. The alphabet was occupied only up to F so there was ample time to eliminate 'P' without causing trouble if its vitamin nature became disproved."

Vitamin P was eventually proven to be bioflavonoids and isoflavonoids, new "co-factors" that were integral parts of the vitamin C complex. In other words, Szent-Györgyi said, without "co-factors" like bioflavonoids and isoflavonoids, you don't have vitamin C, yet when publications like *Time* magazine announced that vitamin C had been "isolated" in the laboratory, the public thought ascorbic acid carried all the healthful qualities that vitamin C contained in an orange, for instance.

Szent-Györgyi contended that human physiology will distinguish the difference between an orange and ascorbic acid blended with bioflavonoids. We may cheat each other in real life, but we can't cheat our bodies, which is the good thing about nature.

Szent-Györgyi realized that bioflavonoids were the transport system that took vitamin C to the actual receptor sites in the body. In other words, the Hungarian biochemist found out that hexuronic acid, or ascorbic acid, by itself, was not a useful compound unless it had the messenger to take the message to the receptor site. What was the messenger? The bioflavonoids in food-created vitamin C.

What Szent-Györgyi didn't know at the time was that he had taken the first step toward unlocking the Vitamin Code. But war clouds were gathering over Europe, and while he was able to continue his work at the University of Szeged, he said that "my democratic ideas brought me more and more into conflict with the rising tide of fascism." During World War II, he was deeply involved in Hungary's resistance movement, working to help Jewish scientists escape the death camps and ferrying messages to the British Secret Service while giving a lecture in Istanbul in the middle of the war.

Upon his return to Hungary, word of his secret mission to Istanbul leaked out. He was placed under house arrest, and then Hitler demanded his delivery. "Arrest would have meant a painful death," he wrote.

Since he expected to be killed, he gathered up his latest research papers and work and left them with friends. Then he went into hiding at the Swedish Legation in Budapest, trading on friendships in the scientific community. A visiting German diplomat, sympathetic to Szent-Györgyi's plight, told him that the Gestapo had searched the surrounding houses for subterranean tunnels to the Swedish Legation and were poised to storm the building at any moment. That night, Per Anger, the head of the Legation, smuggled Szent-Györgyi out in the trunk of his car. Hours later, the Nazis broke into the Swedish Legation and trashed the place in search of Szent-Györgyi. The Hungarian scientist took refuge with friends; bombs destroyed two of his hiding places after he left them. Szent-Györgyi said he avoided arrest by hiding near the Soviet lines where the Gestapo dared not enter.

After the war, the Soviet Union took over Hungary as the

Iron Curtain slammed shut the divide between the East and the West. Szent-Györgyi hoped to be part of rebuilding devastated Hungary by opening a scientific academy for biochemical research. Initially, the Soviet apparatchiks running Hungary cooperated, but as the tentacles of communism squeezed the life out of the Hungarian citizens, Szent-Györgyi sought a way out. The opportunity presented itself while he was on a ski holiday in Switzerland in 1947. He and his wife, Marta, defected and eventually immigrated to the United States, where they settled in Woods Hole, Massachusetts. Szent-Györgyi continued his pioneering research until his death in 1986.

FOLLOWING IN HIS FOOTSTEPS

Paying close attention to Szent-Györgyi's astonishing discoveries with vitamin C was another Hungarian, Endre Szalay, who was seventeen years old when Szent-Györgyi received the Nobel Prize in 1937. The young man, who was vastly interested in science, viewed Szent-Györgyi as a national hero. Two years later in 1939, he enrolled at the University of Szeged in the study of pharmacy, the same institution of higher learning where Szent-Györgyi taught classes and conducted research.

Although their lives would intersect on a minor scale, little did Endre Szalay know that Szent-Györgyi's isolation of vitamin C would lead him down a path that would create a form of nutrients that emulated natural food.

In other words, Endre Szalay would break the Vitamin Code, but it would take him more than three decades to do so, as you'll learn in our next chapter.

Most people, when told it will take decades to unravel a scientific mystery, uncover a cure for a dreaded disease, climb Mount Everest, or—you fill in the blank—would quit long before they reached their objective. It's human nature to focus on the short-term solution rather than the long-term goal.

Endre Szalay never lost sight of where he wanted to go, the frontiers he wanted to explore, or what it would take to get there. To understand why he persevered so long, why he never let go of the dream, you need to hear a story that makes Albert Szent-Györgyi's escape from the Gestapo's clutches sound like a warm-up act.

Break the Code

- Our modern-day diets—heavy on salty snacks, fast food burgers and fries, deep-dish pizza, and sugary desserts—don't provide enough essential vitamins and minerals necessary for optimal health.

- The discovery of various vitamins and minerals in our foods is only a century old, which set off a scientific chase to match those vitamins and minerals in the laboratory.

- Beginning in the 1930s, biochemists such as Albert Szent-Györgyi of Hungary successfully "isolated" various vitamins, such as vitamin C. This led to the development of commercially made vitamins and minerals, which today is a $22 billion annual business.

- Billion-dollar vitamin companies understand that when it comes to sales, the sizzle is more important than the steak. Executives understand that brilliantly executed marketing campaigns and producing the vitamins as cheaply as possible are the ingredients for financial success.

For more information on the world of vitamins and minerals, or to find out more about The Vitamin Code, visit us online at **www.TheVitaminCode.com.**

THE VITΛMIN CODE™

PART 2

CRACKING THE CODE

ENDRE "ANDY" SZΛLΛY
IN HIS OWN WORDS

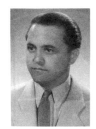

My story begins in Kunszentmiklos, Hungary, where I was born on January 18, 1920. I have lived a long life, eighty-eight years in fact.

Kunszentmiklos is forty miles south of Budapest, and when I was a boy, there were 9,000 inhabitants with a high school of around 400 students. My father taught history and philosophy in middle school; my mother stayed home to raise three active boys. We had our chores around the house, and we were disciplined kids who always wanted to get out of discipline growing up. I was the youngest, so I was my mother's boy. As a spoiled kid, I was always getting in all sorts of trouble. My parents tried to keep me in line with an occasional spanking.

Growing up in Hungary in the 1920s were very, very hard times. Hungary was the loser after the Great War, or what is now called World War I. Thank goodness we always had enough to eat. Both my older brothers were heavily involved in sports. My middle brother was a champion swimmer, so my favorite sport became swimming. I started training when I was ten; my specialty was the freestyle and the backstroke. As I got older, I would swim all summer from 6 until 8 a.m. in the morning, go to school the rest of the day, and then swim from 6 to 8 p.m. in the evening.

High school started at age ten in our system and lasted eight years. Greek or Latin classes were mandatory; I chose Latin for seven years. I can say that I was one of the best in my class. I also took some English classes, but our English teacher was a Hungarian who visited England once in his life for two weeks. He couldn't pronounce a word of English, and I didn't learn a thing.

When I finished high school in the early summer of 1939, war weighed heavily on everyone's mind. Everybody was talking about Germany and Adolf Hitler. I did not know what to do. At that time, being nineteen years old, I had to go into the military service, which was mandatory.

During my medical examination, doctors told me I was half deaf in my left ear, so they did not take me into the army. To this day, I don't know how fortunate I was. My parents had some friends who owned the local pharmacy in town, and they said to me, "Why don't you try to get an education in pharmacy?"

I liked their idea. They directed me to apply to one of the

two pharmacy schools in Hungary. One was at the University of Budapest; the other was at the University of Szeged. I liked Szeged, which had a half-million people. Smaller than Budapest, which had something like 1.5 million people.

I began pharmacy school on September 1, 1939—the same day the Nazi blitzkrieg stormed into Poland. This was an in auspicious beginning as there was tremendous upheaval. Hundreds of thousands, if not millions, of Polish people ran for their lives in the direction of Hungary. Then we started seeing Polish military officers flee into Hungary because word got out that the Germans were executing any officers they captured. This was a trying period.

I signed up to live in a dormitory, but there were some problems, so I decided to live at the Bishop's Palace near the University of Szeged since I was raised Roman Catholic. My friends played a good trick on me, though. When you applied for a room, which was run like a convent, you had to visit the Bishop first. This was a very big deal. My friends told me that I had to be on my best behavior, and if I wanted to get into the Bishop's good graces, I should approach him only on my knees and kiss his ring.

When the door opened to his office, I instantly flung myself to the ground and started walking toward the Bishop on my knees. The Bishop got big eyes and thought this must be a very religious guy. He signaled me to stand up and come to him. I immediately kissed his ring, but he did not let go of my hand. He questioned me for three or four minutes on my family situation, then finally let my hand go. The Bishop approved my request to live there.

The Bishop's Palace was run like a medieval monastery. Every morning—very early—I had to go to the chapel and pray. Every evening before dinner I had to go to the chapel and pray. Every evening after dinner I had to go to the chapel and pray. I could take it only for a month. My roommate and I found a Jewish widow who rented us a room.

I had Jewish friends who were transported to the camps. We didn't know exactly what was happening to the Jews, but we knew it couldn't be good. The Hungarian politicians played very good games with the Germans to keep them from marching into Hungary. We had to send them a lot of food—Hungary was a tremendous agricultural state at the time—as well as hundreds of thousands of Hungarian men to fight with the Nazis on the Russian Front. That's another reason I'm so fortunate to have never been in the army because I would have ended up in Russia. My older brothers weren't so fortunate. My middle brother, an infantryman, was captured by the Russians and spent six years in

Russian camps. My oldest brother was a pilot in the Hungarian Air Force until one day he crashed, burned, and died.

I want to tell you that Hungary was never ready for the war. We were a small country in the middle of Europe. A popular joke at the time went like this: *Germany sent Hungary a message: Send all of your planes to Germany. And Hungary sent Germany a message: Do you want us to send one, or do you want us to send both of them?* Eventually, the Germans did take over, and we did not resist.

Meanwhile, I continued my studies at the University of Szeged. Frequently I saw a gentleman on a bicycle, just riding by. Everyone knew that he was a respected man, this professor. His name was Albert Szent-Györgyi.

You don't know Hungary. We were an old-fashioned country. A professor was either supposed to go to school by car or by a horse-drawn buggy. Szent-Györgyi was the only one who got around with a bicycle. He had long regular pants, but the pants were folded back at the knee, British style. That was because we heard he got his doctorate at Cambridge University.

Here was this famous professor who won the Nobel Prize, riding around on a bicycle when other professors walked around with their noses in the air. He even played soccer with his students, although I never played with him. I never took a class from him, either, but I did visit about ten of his lectures. He wasn't dynamic . . . he was more down-to-earth. He wanted to make the course material so simple so that everyone around him could understand. He was a remarkable man who had quite an effect on me.

I got my pharmacy degree in 1943 and took a job with a pharmacy owned by a friend's family in a village called Rackeve in the middle of an island on the Danube River, not far from Budapest. This was the most horrifying time of my life, when the Russians advanced on Hungary in 1944. The situation deteriorated when the Russians were on the north bank of the Danube, and the Germans were on the south bank. We were trapped in the middle, and the bombing went on for weeks. Such a bombardment, day by day. The Russians were pushing, and the Germans wanted to stop them at the Danube. We hid in the basement until the Russians came into town. We didn't have too many problems with the Germans, but the Russians wanted everything. They robbed the city naked. When they would come into my pharmacy, I couldn't communicate with them, but they certainly made me understand what they wanted. They would rub their stomachs if they had a stomach ache, things like that. After I gave them what they wanted, they walked out without paying.

You cannot imagine what poor condition these Russian soldiers were in when they had already fought the Germans step by step, coming from Stalingrad for thousands of miles. Ten times they pointed a rifle at me and told me what they wanted in the store.I saw the Russians shoot people for nothing—just for looking at them on the street. We lived in great fear.

The Germans were still pounding our village with heavy artillery. One day, a shell hit the top of the pharmacy, and the roof crashed in. I was lucky not to be in the pharmacy at that time, but I had to help cover up the big hole. I got up there with a ladder and put a canvas over the hole, but as I was coming down, I fell and broke my ankle.

Exactly at that time, a doctor was walking by—a doctor I knew. He asked me if everything was all right, but it wasn't. I had broken my ankle pretty badly. He took two or three slices of wood and bandaged me up. That's all he could do. That night, I was in tremendous pain, so my friend gave me a little morphine. Two days later came the order for every civilian to evacuate the town. I had a broken ankle, but that didn't matter. Everyone had to go that night, and it was snowing heavily.

It was a scene right out of the movie, *Dr. Zhivago*—thousands of refugees moving through the snow, walking with what they could carry. I trudged through the snow with a crutch for six kilometers, or four miles, to the next town. I managed to find a room, but not much heat.

The Hungarian men wanted to hide their wives and their daughters because of rape. That was the worst. You could hear the screaming all over the place. There was a woman who used to work with me in the pharmacy, and her family had a chicken in the courtyard. She cut the neck of the chicken, and then this woman wiped the blood on herself.

A Russian soldier insisted on taking her. When she showed the Russian soldier the blood, he decided to move on. She wasn't raped that day, but the humiliation! This is the kind of situation we had over there.

When it was safe to go back to Rackeve, we found out that the Russians had taken every piece of clothing they could find. Some Hungarians had hidden their clothing in the attic or under the roof, but the Russians found these clothes with their search dogs. The Russians then sent the clothes back to Mother Russia because they had nothing, and they were freezing.

We tried to get the pharmacy going again, but the closest supplies were in Budapest, around forty kilometers or twenty-five miles away. My colleague and I borrowed two horses and a wagon, and we collected some food from the local farmers, and put it on the wagon. Then we rode the wagon to Budapest, which didn't have any food. It took eight hours to get there. We went to the supply houses and traded the food for drugs and pharmaceutical items. We must have done twenty trips, but there were people walking on the road, asking if they could hitch a ride on the wagon. We always welcomed them onboard. Sometimes, however, Russian soldiers intercepted us and took all of our food.

Eventually, the Russians moved on to capture Germany. The pharmacy started to come back to life as the war came to an end in Europe. One day, a beautiful girl came into the pharmacy, and being a bachelor, I started to talk to her. She was a pretty one. After talking to her quite a few times, I began pursuing her. Friderike (Frida) and I fell in love, and we got married on September 10, 1946. We did not have a honeymoon. We were so poor. She had lost everything when we had to leave Rackeve, and I had nothing. Between us, we had two sets of clothes. But we had food because many people bartered medicine for eggs, chickens, and vegetables.

After we were married about one or two years, we started to get restless. Let's face it: there was no future for me to work as a pharmacist for someone else. I needed my own pharmacy. I heard about a pharmacy in Budapest where the Jewish owner did not come back, so I rented it from the widow. It included

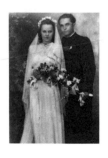

an apartment next door to the pharmacy. Frida gave birth to our two daughters, and we started to have a good life. We were middle class. I became a respected person. In Hungarian culture, we say the priest, the doctor, and the pharmacist are dealing with God.

In the early 1950s, the Communists who took over Hungary started to solidify their grip. They were totalitarians and merciless. They started to nationalize the banks, then other institutions, like big factories, and then they said that in Hungary the pharmacist is a very rich man.

One day, four government Communist Party officials walked into my pharmacy and said, "We are nationalizing. Here is the pen. Take everything out of your pockets, put it on the table, and leave." There was no compensation. I had to hand over my pharmacy that very minute.

One Communist Party official wasn't done. He handed me a piece of paper with an address. "Tomorrow, go to this address and report there because pharmacists are needed in Budapest. We are in short supply, so they will find you a job somewhere. You will become an employee of the state."

Instead of working for the state at the pharmacy next door to my home, however, I was forced to ride a bus two hours one way to manage a pharmacy in another part of Budapest.

The Communists brought in someone else to run my pharmacy. They didn't want me to stay because I knew people and could give them a deal or make a trade.

In those days, there was a lot of handwork in the pharmacy. We did not have everything in a capsule or tablet form like they do now. The doctor would write out what components to put together, and then you would put it all together by hand.

One time I devised a way to make suppositories in a way that you always came out with suppositories the same exact length. Soon, my idea was adopted by 230 other pharmacies in Budapest, and the Communists asked me to visit them, show them how to make the suppositories correctly, things like that. That became my new full-time job, and eventually I was put in charge of eighty-two people. You could say that I was a respected person again at the age of thirty-five.

In the "worker's paradise" in the Communist system, however, this was tantamount to having a bull's eye on your back. You never knew who could say something wrong about you. Happens once—and that's it. They take you away. Maybe for years. You always had this threat hanging over you. All it took was one person denouncing you. I looked around and noticed that everyone with a higher education was gone. I had a university education, which was a huge strike against me. And there was no chance that my two daughters would ever have a higher education.

This was always on my mind, and Frida's, too. We decided that at the first chance, we would get out of the country and start over again. Only better things can come.

We were careful discussing this with each other. We couldn't talk about leaving when we were inside the apartment because we never knew if somebody might be listening in. If the girls—they were nine and eight years old—heard us talking about leaving, they might tell other kids, who would tell their parents. The only time we talked about this possibility was when we sat on a park bench with no one around.

This was a very, very hard decision to make, but we decided to escape from Hungary if the opportunity presented itself. At that time, my mother-in-law was living near the western border, only three kilometers from Austria. If you were caught within one kilometer of the border, they shot you. We visited her to check out how we could escape into Austria anyway.

Three weeks later, out of the blue, the Hungarian Revolution started. On Radio Free Europe, we heard that people were getting out of the country. Twenty one day. One hundred the next. Two-hundred and fifty the day after. I was making my rounds at the pharmacies when a fellow told me, "Did you know the police were here looking for you?"

I got white as a sheet. Somebody had said something about me.

I went home and told Frida what happened. "I have to go," I said, "whether you come with me or not."

"Of course, I come with you," she said. "Children, too."

We left our house the next day with no suitcases, nothing in our hands. Just what we were wearing, like we were going to the park. The neighbors could not think that we were leaving. We got a ride on a truck with thirty other Hungarians to the border, but first we stopped at my mother-in-law's house.

"I'm so happy you came because I was worried that you might miss this chance," she said. Frida's mother said that she had approached the Austrian frontier to check things out. The border patrol—these were Hungarian kids—knew there was a rebellion going on Budapest and didn't know what to do. Meanwhile, people were dashing across the border in droves—too many to shoot.

At the border, a young Hungarian guard said to my mother-in-law, "Why are you here?"

"My family. They want to get out."

"I am here for two more hours. If they come, I will let them through."

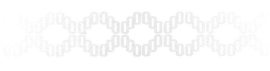

PART 2 — CRACKING THE CODE

This poor old woman, sixty years old, ran back to the house with the incredible news. But we didn't have much time.

My wife and my two kids started walking, and my mother-in-law accompanied us so that she could point out the border guard who said it was okay to escape. He showed us where the land was drier and where there was a hole in the barbwire fence.

Frida and I stepped through with the kids, and then we looked back to her mom. She was weeping because she feared she would never see us again. We were crying, too, because the pain of leaving was unbearable.

"Come over!" Frida said. "Come with us."

In a split second, my mother-in-law stepped through the hole in the fence and joined us. She left everything behind, including her house. At two o'clock in the afternoon on November 18, 1956—a day I will never forget—we were free. Sure, we had only the clothes on our backs, but there wasn't much to take anyway. Even if you had a little money, you couldn't buy clothes in Hungary; none were available in the shops. But in the West, we heard if you work, you can buy clothes.

The Austrian people were wonderful to us. Some of them took us to the mayor's house, where they had food and drink available to us. I had not seen so much food and wine in years. The first night they put us in a refugee camp, which had horrible conditions, but at least we had a roof. The next day, wonders started to happen.

A Catholic priest from the United States, but of Hungarian heritage, took an interest in our family. He asked us where we wanted to go. I said we don't have any money, so what could we do?

"You don't need money," said the priest. "We'll take you wherever you want to go."

We started talking about going to the United States of America. America—where the streets were paved in gold and the lampposts were made with chocolate. Eventually, we were driven to Vienna, where the U.S. Consulate was stationed, and we were given visas to immigrate to the United States. We stayed in another refugee camp for a couple of weeks before we boarded a flight from Vienna to Idlewild airport in New York City, which is known as John F. Kennedy Airport today. We had never been aboard an airplane before, and the prop plane took over twenty-four hours as it made a half-dozen refueling stops along the way, including Prestwick, Scotland; Shannon, Ireland; Reykjavik, Iceland; and Gander, Newfoundland.

Our family and the other refugees on the flight were put into abandoned army barracks in New Jersey. Eventually, I got my first job as a quality control person at a pharmaceutical company. I spoke no English; I only got the job because the boss was Hungarian or knew Hungarian. My American co-workers helped me learn English and make the right pronunciations. Every day, I had to pronounce a new word.

Our little family moved into a cramped apartment. We had linoleum floors; we never had that in Hungary. But we were starting from scratch, and every penny counted. In fact, one morning, I looked all over the house for enough money to pay the bus fare to go to work. All I could find was 18 cents, but the bus fare was 19 cents.

Not knowing what to do, I started walking for the bus stop, and then there it was—a penny on the ground.

When I stooped over to pick up that penny, I knew I was going to be all right, and so was my family.

△   △   △

Wasn't that a wonderful story? I (Massoud) have known Andy for nearly twenty years, but he has never told anyone—and I mean anyone, including his daughters—the story you just read. But now that he's in the autumn years of his life, he feels a need to share his compelling life story so that his subsequent scientific discoveries will give you some perspective about where he is coming from, to use a particularly American phrase.

In early 1957, his first job with a botanical company was what we call a "bench chemist," which was the lowest job available for someone with a pharmacist background. No one paid attention to him because his pharmacy degree—which had a heavy emphasis in pharmacognostica and chemistry—was from Hungary. (Pharmacognosy is a multidisciplinary subject that comprises parts of botany, organic chemistry, biochemistry, pharmacology, zoology, anthropology, geography, ethnomedicine, nutraceuticals, and medicinal plants. Pharmacognosy is the oldest medical science, a counterpart to the study of medicine since early pharmacognosists were physicians.)

Basically, Andy was a lowly technician in a company laboratory. As he learned English and gained confidence, though, he began contributing in amazing ways. He discovered more active ingredients in various herbs and devised more efficient ways to purify and crystallize many of these active ingredients.

For the next twenty years, Andy worked for three botanical/pharmaceutical companies in the northeast corner of New Jersey, Bergen County, where Manhattan and New York City lay across the Hudson River. The family settled in the leafy town of Hackensack, New Jersey, and though the lampposts weren't made with chocolate, the girls quickly adapted to their new lives in the United States.

Andy became a poster boy for the American Dream. At all three companies, he climbed the ladder so quickly that at his last job, he was named vice president and was basically running the day-to-day operations. The best research-and-development ideas came from him, the laboratory work was supervised by him, and dozens of employees and departments reported directly to him. Everyone appreciated his pioneering ideas and the products he came up with, and once again—just as in Budapest—he had earned respect. It was a meteoric rise when you consider his humble arrival in the United States and his lack of English language skills.

Every year or two, however, he would tell his bosses that he had a great idea that he wanted to explore—an idea that stemmed from his youngest days when he studied biochemistry at the University of Szeged. No one paid attention to him, even though the companies he worked for were doing very well financially because of his superior intellect and stellar abilities in the research laboratory.

Andy was convinced that food contained the most amazing, and, of course, the most nutritious compounds in the world, yet as he looked around in the 1950s, 1960s, and 1970s, huge pharmaceutical firms were introducing and successfully marketing nutritional supplements produced from synthetic, laboratory-derived materials. Common sense and Albert Szent-Györgyi's work told him otherwise. Regarding the former, Andy knew that human physiology will distinguish the difference between the vitamin C in an orange and ascorbic acid isolated from paprika or synthetically manufactured in a laboratory. As for Szent-Györgyi, he had discovered that an "intermediary" form of ascorbic acid—one that resembled food without the bulk of the food—was more successful at curing scurvy in laboratory animals than the pure, crystalline form of ascorbic acid that had gone through many steps of isolation and purification.

Swimming against the prevailing tide, Andy believed that if these synthetically made nutrients could somehow be brought back to their natural form, they would match the nutritive power found in real food. No one wanted to hear Andy's theories, however. Perhaps that's because the conventional wisdom in the 1970s proclaimed that "mega-dosing"—taking vitamins and minerals in amounts way beyond recommended daily values opened the gateway to good health. The floodgates were thrust apart by Linus Pauling, Ph.D., who wrote a revolutionary book in 1970 called *Vitamin C and the Common Cold*. In his best-selling book that paid homage to Albert Szent-Györgyi's pioneering work, Dr. Pauling postulated that taking 1,000 milligrams of vitamin C daily could bolster the immune system for most people.

A thousand milligrams (or 1 gram) happened to be a massive amount of vitamin C because the U.S. government's recommended daily allowance (RDA) was only 60 mg.

Suddenly, everyone was talking about the "miracle" of vitamin C. After the mainstream media—*New York Times, Newsweek, Reader's Digest*—jumped on the bandwagon and spread the gospel of vitamin C megatherapy, people in the '70s gulped vitamin C tablets like kids reaching for a bowl of M&Ms. Andy, however, was sure our bodies were not designed to consume these supplements in such enormous quantities. When he heard that some people were taking as many as ten 1,000-miligram tablets of vitamin C, he knew that this was the equivalent of eating fifty to one hundred oranges in a single day. Talk about a colon cleanse: diarrhea, abdominal cramps, and nausea were among the common side effects of vitamin C megadosing. Andy felt that the only reason to take vitamins and minerals by the handful was precisely because they *were* synthetic, isolated products that delivered very little of nature's nutrients to the body.

Synthetic versions of vitamin C or most other nutrients on the market were not really vitamins and minerals—they were *precursors,* or a substance that preceded another substance. In other words, ascorbic acid was a precursor to the vitamin C found in citrus fruits and would never match up to the real deal. That's why Andy believed that health-minded individuals had to go back to *food-created* nutrients if they were interested in supplementing their diets. Was it possible to develop nutrients that came as close to natural food without the bulk of the food? That was the $64,000 question that Andy had wanted to explore ever since he dropped by Szent-Györgyi's lectures at the University of Szeged.

Except that a remarkable life—and the responsibilities to his work and his family—kept getting in the way. By the mid-1970s, Andy had faithfully been at his third company for more than fifteen years. He had risen to vice president in charge of operations and was the driving engine behind the organization's growth and profitability. He thought he would receive company stock or become part owner in recognition of his contributions to the company's profitable bottom line, but when that didn't happen, he began to explore his options.

Although he was fifty-seven years old, he said to himself, "Maybe it's not too late to come up with a new discovery." What he really wanted to do was study and evaluate what the active stage was for every individual nutrient—and develop vitamins and minerals that were as close to natural food as possible. Like the day he and his family stepped through a hole in the barbwire at the Austrian border and entered the Great Unknown, Andy risked everything by leaving the job that he had always assumed to be his last professional position to start his own company in 1977. Within two weeks, he leased a small office and manufacturing plant near his hometown of Hackensack and hung out a shingle for a corporation that he called the Grow Company.

Because of Andy's superior people skills, he had developed great relationships with suppliers and customers. Many of them had encouraged him to strike out on his own. They granted him credit purely on the trust he had developed with them over the years. He initially hired five employees—people he had worked with, one way or another, over the last twenty years. When Andy informed some prospective hires that he couldn't take them aboard just yet because he didn't have money to pay them, they said they'd come to work for Grow Company anyway. "When you make money, you can pay us at that time," they said.

Andy couldn't let that happen, so he dipped into his dwindling personal savings accounts to make payroll each week. He made his first sale—a blend of different herbs—within two or three months and slowly built up a customer base. As business grew and he had people to delegate work to, Andy turned his energies toward developing the first food-created vitamins and minerals, a process that would eventually crack the Vitamin Code.

THE EUREK∆ MOMENT

At first, Andy's idea was to buy a large parcel of New Jersey farmland—hundreds of acres—and raise organic vegetables and fruits that he could harvest, dehydrate, then mill, extract, concentrate, and tablet the resultant natural food concentrate. Throughout the process, he would be checking for ways to improve the potency of the active ingredients as well as research the active stages of each individual nutrient found in these foods.

As he thought through this idea, Andy realized that it would take a tremendous amount of land to plant all the foods needed to create the broad array of nutrients that were needed. In addition, New Jersey farmland was sure to harbor environmental problems. The Garden State was called the "Garbage State" by detractors because of upwards of 16,000 contaminated sites in the state, ranging from minor leaks at residential heating oil tanks to Superfund sites. The state's contaminated areas included old factories, some possibly with radioactive waste, petroleum byproducts, and toxic solvents.

So Andy realized that farms were not the answer and turned his attention back to studying the active ingredients in fruits and vegetables. He knew that plant roots picked up inorganic mineral salts from the soil, brought them up through the trunk, and then moved them to the stems and eventually to the leaves or fruit. When the sun shines on a plant, the whole metabolic condition comes alive; the leaves and fruit come out, and *voilà*, you have vitamins and minerals in spades. In other words, nature converted the inorganic salts in the soil to organic entities in the leaves and fruit, which became the delivery agents for the vitamin and mineral nutrients.

Plants, as Andy had learned back in high school biology in the 1930s, were multi-cell organisms—and vastly complicated. An idea began to percolate: What if he backed down to a simple single-cell plant or microorganism and explored the possibilities with this source? The most popular single-cell plant was yeast; in fact, there were a few hundred genomes of yeast available in the world. The best single-cell yeast Andy could find was *Saccharomyces cerevisiae*, the Latin name for baker's yeast, a common household ingredient found in nearly every pantry. Everyone with a bread machine knows that when you bake bread, you pour in water and olive oil, the requisite flour and salt, add yeast, and turn on the machine, which slowly churns the dough and makes the mixture active. The yeast starts growing and budding, causing the dough to rise. When the bread dough is baked, the yeast is deactivated.

When Andy began experimenting with baker's yeast in the laboratory, he realized that he could control everything. He could control the environment. He could control how fast he wanted to grow the yeast. He could control how long the yeast was going to be live and active, and he could control what he fed the yeast. If he had pursued the idea of buying New Jersey farmland, his best-case scenario was reaping two or three crops a year, but with baker's yeast, he could bring it to life any day he wanted to, or he could deactivate and harvest it whenever he desired. Nor was he limited to the weather because he could plant and grow these single-cell microorganisms hydroponically—meaning in water.

Plants receive their nutrients from the soil. Single-cell organisms like baker's yeast grown hydroponically take whatever nutrient is in an absorbable form from the water and metabolize it inside its cells. Yeast, when brought to life, starts budding and then propagating, which means the single cell goes from one cell to two cells, two cells split into four cells, four cells into sixteen cells, and so forth. Andy put yeast in reactors, added water, fed the yeast with nutrients, and watched yeast come to life—just like a fruit tree in an orchard.

What Andy discovered is that when yeast comes to life and

he fed the yeast with nutrients in their appropriate form, the nutrients traveled through the cell walls of the yeast and reacted with the protein of the yeast. Once the reaction with the protein of the yeast occurred, it became part of the yeast. Yeast, by nature, has B vitamins, vitamin D, plus minerals, which are in appropriate or "replaceable" receptor sites in the yeast. What Andy ascertained through trial and error was that there were empty receptor sites in the yeast—empty sites that could be filled by the addition of various nutrients. Eventually, Andy learned he could "feed" the yeast with proteins and peptides—combined and linked amino acids—because they could penetrate through the cells walls. Proteins and peptides did not need a passport or visa to go through the cell walls. They could get inside the cell with only the yeast cells' permission.

Over a period of several years, through unbelievable trial and error, Andy figured out that he could take vitamins and minerals—such as thiamine (B1) or calcium—and embed them into those proteins and peptides, then introduce the result into the budding, growing, and propagating single-cell *Saccharomyces cerevisiae*, or baker's yeast.

This meant that a concentrated form of vitamin or mineral was fed back into a food medium in which that vitamin or mineral would naturally be found. The complex then undergoes a growth and/or activation process that results in the vitamin or mineral being integrated into the food matrix in the same way it would be found naturally.

Andy was getting closer to unlocking the Vitamin Code. He conducted dozens of more experiments, approximately fifty or sixty trials for each nutrient, and came upon a concentrate—later called Code Factors—that was inherent to each specific nutrient. Upon discovery of the Code Factors, he devised a protocol to metabolize the nutrient in a budding and propagating single-cell baker's yeast.

When Andy added thiamine hydrochloride (B1) and fed it to the baker's yeast, the yeast metabolized the thiamine and converted it into a food-created nutrient that was, for all intents and purposes, the real version of thiamine. In nature, thiamine is not associated with hydrochloric acid to generate a salt of thiamine, but it is in the free form of thiamine. In other words, Andy had figured out a way to reverse-engineer the work of Albert Szent-Györgyi because he could take a substance like ascorbic acid and turn it back into the "original" vitamin C found in its more natural state, with its "co-factors" intact.

This was the "Eureka!" moment. But how did Andy know that

this yeast with metabolized vitamins and minerals inside the cell and/or on the cell walls was any better than vitamins and minerals produced synthetically? The first thing Andy did was commission an outside laboratory to check every batch to make sure it wasn't toxic. Lo and behold, many of his original plant trials with *Saccharomyces cerevisiae*, or baker's yeast, were indeed toxic. Although he didn't have to go back to the drawing board, it took Andy several more years figuring out the right parameters to produce toxic-free nutrients from baker's yeast.

After he could set aside the toxicity concerns, Andy turned his attention toward the efficacy of his newly formulated products. Again, batches were shipped to outside, third-party university laboratories for comparison to other nutrients. What efficacy did these products have? Eventually, research scientists formed the opinion that these products were a new breed of nutrients but with an inherent ancient wisdom that made them as close to food as possible.

Andy Szalay, the Hungarian immigrant who had come to this country with no money in his pocket, had cracked the Vitamin Code.

Or had he? In Andy's mind, he was certain that he discovered a blueprint that he could use to manufacture every nutrient in the universe, but as he created more test batches in the laboratory, he discovered that he had been completely wrong. The blueprint of one vitamin or one mineral was not applicable to another vitamin or mineral. Every nutrient has its own blueprint, its own fingerprint, which is why it took even more years of testing to complete the set and come up with whole spectrum of nutrients in the form of food.

His first success was with a mineral called selenium. Selenium is an essential trace mineral, and only a small amount is necessary to obtain the benefits. Selenium is incorporated into proteins to make selenoproteins, which are important antioxidant enzymes that help prevent cellular damage from free radicals. Free radicals are natural byproducts of oxygen metabolism that may contribute to the development of health problems. Other selenoproteins support healthy thyroid function and promote a healthy immune system.

Andy took selenium, embedded it in the proper peptide, and fed it to the yeast. The peptide went through the cell walls, which means the selenium was now inside the cell. What Andy was discovering was that in nature, 1 + 1 was not 2. In this instance, 1 + 1 went way beyond 2—synergy!

That was the beauty of breaking the Vitamin Code, creating nutrient-enhanced yeast and other food products that had undergone a unique activation and growth process. The result was the creation of whole food ingredients where the enhanced level of nutrients formed an integral part of the yeast and other Code Factors in an organic food complex.

PRACTICAL APPLICATIONS

What I (Massoud) have described to you is what Andy was doing between the years of 1977 and 1990. As news of Andy's exciting work spread through the biochemist grapevine, pharmaceutical companies, food companies, and cosmetic companies started their evaluation process of Andy's breakthroughs and began coming up with practical applications in the marketplace. For instance, commercial bakeries realized that by adding Andy's food created nutrients to carrot cake, they could increase the shelf life of that product.

You may be too young to remember this, but ten, twenty years ago, supermarkets and bakeries had to sell their carrot cakes within two or three days, after which spoilage set in. (Carrots quickly deteriorate.) With Andy's food created nutrients, however, carrot cake remains fresh longer on the store shelf, which gives the cake a huge sales advantage.

These days, there's a strong chance that the carrot cake you see in the warehouse club or supermarket has benefited from Andy's diligence in breaking the Vitamin Code. Other foods such as sushi, gelatin, baked goods, and Asian foods benefited from the same application of these nutrients, which improved their taste, fortified the food, and acted as a flavoring or natural coloring agent.

These applications have been making their way into the marketplace since the early 1980s, when Grow Company began making them available to manufacturers From the first day, though, Andy decided that Grow Company would never distribute its products to the end user. Instead, entrepreneurially minded companies could purchase various Grow Company nutrients manufactured at the Ridgefield plant and use them in their field of business as they best saw fit.

One of those future-minded companies was Garden of Life, based in West Palm Beach, Florida. When the company founder, Jordan Rubin learned that Grow Company's food-created nutrients could be used to produce novel, high-quality nutritional supplements, they began a dialogue with me about telling the world how Andy cracked the so-called "vitamin code."

As the vice president of Grow Company and responsible for the day-to-day operations while Andy, eighty-eight years young, enjoys the fruits of semi-retirement, I believed the partnership would benefit both sides. In 2008, Garden of Life introduced a new line of vitamin and mineral supplements called "raw food-created" nutrients in a unique combination based on Andy's groundbreaking discovery. These multivitamins, which provide nutrients the way nature intended. We believe they are the ultimate in nutritional supplementation.

We'll explain why in our next section as we unpack the commercial side of nutritional supplementation. By the time you finish reading the next part of *The Vitamin Code*, you'll have a greater understanding about why Vitamin Code multivitamins from Garden of Life bring the work of Albert Szent-Györgyi full circle.

Break the Code

- Endre "Andy" Szalay and his family took an incredible risk to escape from behind Iron Curtain during the Hungarian Revolution in 1956, arriving in America with little more than the clothes on their backs.

- Andy believed that commercial vitamins and minerals made from synthetic, isolated sources failed to deliver nature's nutrients to the body, nor was he sold on "megadosing"—taking five, ten times the recommended amount of a certain vitamin or mineral.

- Andy began his experiments with a single-cell yeast called Saccharomyces cerevisiae, and after years of trial and error, discovered how to feed the yeast with nutrients that traveled through the cell walls and became part of the yeast. Feeding the yeast an isolated vitamin like ascorbic acid created a substance that was more closely related to the natural form of vitamin C found in citrus fruits.

- When Andy broke the Vitamin Code, his scientific discoveries had other applications, including adding shelf life to certain foods like carrot cake. But the latest and most important application could be the new line of multivitamins that use raw food-created nutrients.

To learn more about this breakthrough discovery that will change the way you take vitamins forever, visit us online at **www.TheVitaminCode.com.**

PART 3

WHAT THE VITAMIN CODE MEANS FOR YOU

As scientific knowledge progressed throughout the 20th century, an idea took hold that all the nutrients the body would ever need—the essential vitamins and minerals—could be compressed into the size of a capsule. The futuristic cartoon show originating in the 1960s, *The Jetsons*, tapped into this *zeitgeist* by showing Jane Jetson lifting a tureen cover to reveal a colorful array of pills for dinner—pills that simulated the taste and flavor of steak, potatoes, and Pineapple Upside-Down Cake.

These days we know that swallowing a handful of pills—including store-bought vitamins and minerals—can't replace the all-around nutrition found in a healthy meal made from farm-fresh foods. At the same time, though, we believe that we've successfully made the case that we *do* need to supplement our diets because our foods lack nutritional punch. Levels of iron, calcium, and vitamins A and C in our produce, for example, have dropped dramatically since the 1940s. A study published in *August Celebration* found that in 1948, 100 grams of spinach contained 158 milligrams of iron. The same quantity of spinach contains less than 2.2 milligrams of iron today, meaning you'd have to eat seventy-five rations of spinach just to match the same nutritional wallop. I (Massoud) don't like to think of myself as being *that* old, but today's rubbery and flavorless tomatoes can't compare to the ruby-red, sun-ripened, and delicious tomatoes that I picked off the vine as an Iranian youth and ate like a fresh apple.

Perhaps the mealy taste and lack of flavor is why many Americans don't like to eat their fruits and veggies. Instead, our fast-food nation is hooked on greasy burgers and chicken nuggets, captivated by sweets, and relatively clueless about what's healthy to eat. When we do venture into supermarkets these days, many bypass the produce sections and choose to fill their carts with frozen meals or boxed goodies prepared in assembly-line fashion in some faraway factory with zero-nutrient ingredients like refined white flour and refined sugar. Huge food conglomerates add a plethora of additives and preservatives to extend a product's shelf life, which lowers its nutrition ranking from bad to worse. You would have thought that we learned our lesson from Dr. Eijkman, but it's clear that we haven't.

Whatever the reason—processed foods, drive-thru meals, gaps in our diets, or kids who don't like vegetables—millions of Americans like Dawn Saunders purchase vitamin and mineral supplements as an insurance policy to augment the nutrition they receive on a daily basis. When shopping for nutritional supplements, though, it pays to be an informed consumer.

The first thing you need to know is that commercially sold vitamins and minerals are manufactured from different sources that vary widely in their composition, their ingredients, and their quality. We can differentiate nutritional supplements into five separate categories, which are represented in the following pyramid. The very ones in which Andy Szalay discovered by cracking the "vitamin code" form a category that we call Raw Food-Created Nutrients. You'll notice that Raw Food-Created Nutrients are at the top of the pyramid pictured below, representing their innovative qualities:

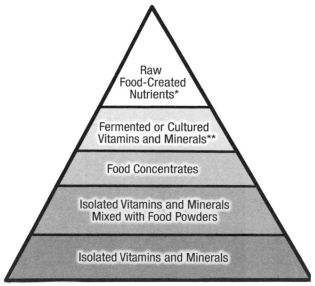

Raw
Food-Created
Nutrients*

Fermented or Cultured
Vitamins and Minerals**

Food Concentrates

Isolated Vitamins and Minerals
Mixed with Food Powders

Isolated Vitamins and Minerals

* Raw Food Created Nutrients include isolated vitamins and minerals that have been renatured (grown) into a form closer to food.

** Fermented or Cultured Vitamins and Minerals include isolated vitamins and minerals that are added to food and herbal concentrates and then fermented with probiotics.

These designations may come across as code words, part of a secret language that everyone else is speaking except for you. Put those concerns aside. Once you understand the distinctions between these five categories, you'll shop with confidence the next time you step inside a health food store or vitamin outlet. Since a further explanation of each category is in order, we'll begin with Isolated Vitamins and Minerals.

ISOLATED VITAMINS AND MINERALS

Isolated multivitamins are the most popular supplements on the market, outselling every other kind of vitamin and mineral on the store shelves. Most vitamins in your supermarket or drug store have a suggested use of "one a day." These days, shoppers are practically programmed to think that taking a multivitamin one time per day will cover their nutritional bases. A typical multivitamin bottle has a box of information printed on the back label called "Supplement Facts."

Scanning through this information, you may be thinking: *Okay, looks like I've got all the important vitamins locked up: A, C, D, and a bunch of B vitamins. A hundred percent of the Recommended Daily Value? Check. Guess I'm covered.*

Not so quick.

Two issues are at play here. First is the RDA, or Recommended Daily Allowance, which is also known as DVs (Daily Values) or DVRs (Daily References Values). The RDA is a U.S. governmental standard that estimates the minimum amount of a nutrient that the body needs to stay healthy. We believe, however, that the use of RDAs fails to adequately address your unique and individual nutritional needs since some of the recommendations are more than thirty years old and have not kept pace with the latest nutritional research. Look at RDAs like minimum-wage jobs: it's barely enough to get by and certainly not enough to thrive. In addition, some companies add insignificant ingredients to make their product's RDA breakdown look more impressive.

The second issue is that the isolated, purified vitamins and minerals are nothing more than synthetic versions of common nutrients like vitamin C, vitamin A, and vitamin E. When vitamins are mass-produced from laboratory-manufactured sources, they are known in the industry as synthetic isolates.

If you'll recall from our opening section, we explained how biochemical scientists in white lab coats have discovered ways to synthetically replicate nutrients in the laboratory. Man's genius—which started with Albert Szent-Györgyi isolating ascorbic acid, or vitamin C, from Hungarian paprika—has devised clever ways to scientifically craft imitations of the real nutrients contained in various foods, but these synthetic versions can never be the same as vitamins and minerals in food form.

So, how can you tell if your multivitamin is filled with synthetic nutrients? The place to start is with the fine print on the label affixed to the back of the bottle or plastic container. If, for example, a bottle of chewable vitamin C tablets lists ingredients such as ascorbic acid, natural or artificial orange flavor, sucralose, or yellow 6 lake, then the product is probably synthetic materials through and through.

Another tip-off is if any of the ingredients have the letters "dl" in front of the name of the vitamin. For instance, if you pick up a bottle of vitamin E and see that the main ingredient is named "dl-alpha tochopheryl," that means you're holding a synthetic version. An ingredient named "d-alpha tochopheryl," however, ("d" instead of "dl") would mean that this is a natural version of vitamin E. Finally, if the label lists many chemical names for various vitamins, such as pyridoxine hydrochloride, thiamin mononitrate, or cholecalciferol, you are holding a vitamin made from synthetic sources.

HERE'S A PARTIAL LIST THAT SHOULD PROVE HELPFUL:

NAME OF VITAMIN	NATURAL	SYNTHETIC
Vitamin A	Fish Oils	Acetate or Palmitate
Vitamin B1	Yeast, Rice Bran	Thiamine Mononitrate, Thiamine Hydrochloride, Thiamine Mononitrate
Vitamin B2	Yeast, Rice Bran	Riboflavin, Riboflavin Monophosphate
Vitamin B3 (or niacin)	Yeast, Rice Bran	Niacinamide, Nicotinamide, Nicotinic Acid Amide
Vitamin B6	Yeast, Rice Bran	Pyridoxine Hydrochloride
Vitamin B12	Yeast, Liver Fermentation	Cobalamin, Cyancobalamin, Methylcobalamin
Vitamin C	Citrus Fruits, Green Peppers, Rose Hips, Acerola, Wildberry	Ascorbic Acid, Ascorbyl Palmitate, Calcium Ascorbate
Vitamin D	Cod Liver Oil or Fish Oil	Irradiated Ergosterol, Calciferol, or Ergocalciferol
Vitamin E	Vegetable Oils, Wheat Germ, or D-Alpha Tocopherol	Dl-Alpha Tocopherol
Vitamin K	Alfalfa	Menadione

A final word of advice regarding isolated, purified vitamins and minerals: stay away from tablet products that come in colorful hues, which generally is a tip off that sugars, artificial sweeteners, artificial colors, and artificial flavorings were used. Nearly all "chewable" vitamins contain high fructose corn syrup, a sugar, to make their taste palatable, especially to young children.

ISOLATED VITAMINS AND MINERALS MIXED WITH FOOD POWDERS

Some vitamin manufacturers add food powders to "improve" their products and give them a marketing edge. You might even see the word "Natural" or "Whole Food" emblazoned on some of the bottles in this category, but keep in mind that the FDA has never defined "natural" or "whole food."

When synthetically derived vitamins and minerals fully dissolve in the body, even when they've been sprinkled with food powder, the physiological processes at work are thrown for a loop, so to speak, because of the shape of the molecules making up the synthetically isolated vitamin or mineral. What happens is these molecules are often the mirror image of their natural counterparts. It's like holding your right hand up to your left hand: they are mirror images of each other, related to be sure, but fundamentally different in the end. (Just try wearing a left-handed golf glove on your right hand.) Synthetic vitamins contain molecules that are left-handed versions of what is found in nature as right-handed molecules. The body doesn't know how to react to their introduction, so the result is ineffectiveness.

We guestimate that more than 99 percent of consumers are unaware of technical information like this, but even if they were, many would continue to purchase vitamins and minerals anyway because of price. When Dawn Saunders shops at her local warehouse club for vitamin C, she can purchase 500 tablets of Vitamin C, 1000 mg with rose hips for only $9.99. Since Dawn has been unaware that ascorbic acid is a synthetic version of vitamin C, why should she pay more for vitamin C produced naturally from concentrated foods in the form of raw food-created nutrients?

The world's major producers of commercial vitamins and minerals know that the public is fixated on buying vitamins as cheaply as possible, unwilling to educate themselves about what's really inside the bottle, and susceptible to flim-flam advertising campaigns. That's why there's little incentive for vitamin makers to change the way they've always done business.

And what a good business it's been for the handful of companies— a dozen or so worldwide—that manufacture the isolated, synthetic ingredients used to make vitamins. We're talking about billion-dollar behemoths that basically run a cartel that matches what the OPEC countries have done with oil. Their global domination has been undercut in the last few years by China, however, because Chinese manufacturers spotted a market ripe for the taking. By 2008, Chinese vitamin manufacturers had grabbed 90 percent of the U.S. market for vitamin C, as well as a majority of vitamins A, B12, and E sold in this country, according to the *Seattle Times*.

For those concerned about the purity of the vitamins they buy, be aware that U.S. laws don't require vitamin manufacturers to label their ingredients with the country of origin, making it impossible for consumers to know where their supplements are coming from.

A Look Behind the Manufacturing of Vitamins

by Massoud Arvanaghi, PhD

The world of supplements and vitamins can be confusing for everyday Americans looking to be healthy, as we have illustrated so far. One aspect that consumers often times overlook is how a product is manufactured, and more importantly, what happens to the "raw material" during that production process.

Although many marketers employ a whole host of novel forms for vitamins and minerals—such as liquid drinks, gummy animals, chocolate chews, or effervescent wafers—the primary options for taking supplements are tablets or capsules.

Tablets are the most popular and widely available option to the consumer. Many people looking for a convenient, once-a-day formula find the tablet ideal for taking their multivitamins. The primary advantage of a tablet is that you are able to compress a relatively large amount of raw material into a compact pill, making it easy to swallow. This convenience, however, comes with a cost.

In order to make a tablet, a surprisingly large amount of steps need to be followed to ensure that the tablet maintains the same shape all the way from the factory floor to your cupboard. Ingredients are mixed, blended, and sometimes ground or pulverized to make sure the particle size of the raw material is consistent. Depending on the raw material that is being tableted, binding agents are added to ensure the material holds together throughout the tableting process.

Just a few decades ago, small mom-and-pop companies would manufacture their products in backyard sheds; today, however, the industry utilizes state-of-the-art facilities, cutting-edge technology, and manufacturing best practices to realize efficiencies, improve quality, and ensure speedier delivery to market. What this means is that practically all the vitamins or supplements you see on a store shelf go through multiple stages in the manufacturing process. In order to automate and streamline the transfer of raw material from one stage and one machine to the next, flow agents are sometimes added to the raw material to allow for the expeditious transfer of ingredients throughout the factory.

When it comes time to compress that raw material into a tablet, a special machine that generates an intense amount of pressure "punches" the material through a mold or die. Unfortunately, it also takes high amounts of heat and pressure to punch the tablet, which can alter or affect the integrity of the raw material. And as manufacturers are always looking to optimize production, they are finding ways to produce more tablets per minute. The fastest tablet machines typically have the highest heat and pressure.

One final step required to ensure the material holds together through the packaging stage and transportation to the marketplace is spray coating. This is yet another step of processing where inactive ingredients or added compounds—also known as fillers— comprise the coating. This process needs high temperatures at the application of the coating and the drying time.

When evaluating the products available on the shelf, look for the term "Other ingredients" on the back of the bottle or packaging. There you will find binders, fillers, excipients, flow agents, and other additives such as:

• **Maltodextrin**	• **Corn Starch**	• **Magnesium Stearate**
• **Stearic Acid**	• **Silica**	• **Cellulose Gum**
• **Guar Gum**	• **Soy Lecith**	• **Milled Soy**

A few of these additives do have some nutritive value, but they are relatively low in comparison to the vitamins, minerals, or other key nutrients you are looking to receive from the product. The percentage of the tablet considered "Other ingredients" is variable, and FDA regulations do not require supplement manufacturers to disclose exactly how much of these "Other ingredients" are in the product. They are only required to list them in descending order.

Besides tablets, consumers can take their supplements in capsule form. Encapsulation fills and combines two ends of a capsule with the raw material ingredients. The primary drawback of this delivery form is that manufacturers can fit less material into the shape size. For instance, one of the largest capsules available will hold approximately 700-750 mg of material, whereas a tablet approximately the same size will hold 1400 mg of material—nearly twice as much.

The advantage of encapsulation, especially when aiming to deliver a raw food-created nutrient, is that there are minimal steps in the process. You don't have the need for binders, fillers, high pressure and heat tableting, or spray coating, so the material maintains its intrinsic value and pristine quality throughout the manufacturing process to bring the product to market.

With the Vitamin Code Raw Food-Created Nutrients, you will find an encapsulated material that has been meticulously controlled and minimally handled to deliver you the highest quality raw food nutrients possible. Vitamin Code formulas are uncooked, untreated, unadulterated, minimally processed, and contain live enzymes and probiotics, delivering to you the ultimate in raw, whole food nutrition.

FOOD CONCENTRATES

We are now entering a stratum of food-based vitamins derived from vegetable, mineral, or animal sources. This initial category—Food Concentrates—are different than isolate-created vitamins. When vitamins and minerals are produced from food-based sources, they are more body-friendly. The next three categories on the pyramid are examples of supplements produced from food-based sources.

Examples would be extracting vitamins A and D from fish liver oil; vitamin E from soy oil; and lecithin from soybeans. Cereal grasses such as barely grass, wheat grass, oat grass, and alfalfa grass contain a broad array of enzymes, vitamins, minerals, proteins, and chlorophyll, which is the green pigment found in plants. Chlorophyll makes life on earth possible because the oxygen we breathe comes from the chlorophyll-rich green plants.

Our human blood is identical to chlorophyll with one exception: the main element in blood is iron, while the main element in chlorophyll is magnesium. The nutritive density found in barley or other grasses such as wheat, rye, corn, rice, oats, sorghum, millet, and spelt is exceptional.

Many of the popular "green food" supplements found today are a blend of barley, wheat, oat, and alfalfa grasses that have had the moisture "dried" out of them and been concentrated into a powder or liquid form. The nutritional content in a high-quality green food powder often has great amounts of various nutrients such as vitamin A, riboflavin, folic acid, magnesium, and calcium. Cereal grass is richer in nutrients than spinach, broccoli, eggs, and chicken in virtually all categories, including protein. Cereal grass abounds in unidentified growth factors, powerful antioxidants, immune boosters, and many other health-supporting nutrients.

Historically, the older school of thought regarding nutritional supplementation dates back to the 1930s, a time when there was an emphasis on the utilization of whole food concentrates as a source of essential nutrients. Before synthetic vitamin supplements were available, concentrated foods such as wheat and barley grass were considered our first "multivitamins." Doctors handed "grass tablets" to patients with nutrient deficiencies or for specific health conditions. Because the vitamin content of cereal grass was much higher than vegetables, they suggested that using cereal grass as a human food supplement would be an economical way to provide the nutrients commonly lacking in the American diet.

The dehydrated cereal grass most commonly used was called Cerophyl (from the Latin word *cerealis*, meaning "of grain," and the Greek word *phyllon*, meaning "leaf"). The Council on Foods of the American Medical Association in fact, approved Cerophyl as an "accepted food" in 1939. The AMA acceptance notice recognized the value of cereal grass not only as a rich source of carotene and vitamin K, but also as a solid source of vitamin C and the B vitamins.

During the 1950s, chemical and pharmaceutical industries began to play a bigger role in the production and delivery of American foods. They heavily promoted the idea that breakthroughs in technology and science could lead to better living, spearheaded with a fertilized, crop sprayed "green revolution." At the same time, agrochemicals began accumulating in our soils and on our crops. Synthetic nutrients were added to foods and also pressed into vitamin pills. As multivitamin pills (synthetic) and vitamin isolates became more commonplace, food-based nutritional supplements such as Cerophyl became less popular.

FERMENTED OR CULTURED VITΛMINS ΛND MINERΛLS

When a living probiotic culture is added to "food concentrated" vitamins and minerals, the result the conversion of one ingredient to another with complete structural change. Fermented or Cultured Vitamins and Minerals, also known as "whole food" vitamins and minerals, start with ingredients that are unprocessed, unrefined, or processed and refined as little as possible. Isolated vitamins and minerals are combined with food and herbal concentrates and undergo a process called "probiotic fermentation." Probiotic fermentation is a process where beneficial bacteria and yeasts convert various compounds to another through a fermentation process, thus creating a "living food" or "living supplement." A simple example of fermentation is the conversion of sugar to alcohol. This is the process where grape juice is converted into a fermented beverage that we know as wine.

Think back to your high school biology class. Everything starts with plant life, and plants get their nutrients through biological transmutation, a process in which soil organisms take inorganic nutrients and convert them into organic substances that can be consumed by humans. Put another way, the microorganisms found in soil and on plants secrete various acids and enzymes to break down inorganic substances and convert them into organic substances that our bodies can use.

Supplements made with concentrated food ingredients and a fermentation process introduce beneficial bacteria in the digestive tract. Many people are not aware that the normal gastrointestinal tract contains hundreds of different species of harmless or even beneficial microorganisms, otherwise known as intestinal flora. Probiotics, which are living, direct-fed microbials (DFMs), promote the growth of beneficial bacterial in the intestines.

In light of Andy's research into baker's yeast or *Saccharomyces cerevisiae*, it's interesting to note that some of the most important microorganisms that the body should receive are probiotics of "friendly" yeasts, such as *Saccharomyces boulardii*, a sub-specie of *Saccharomyces cerevisiae*. Probiotic yeasts have been shown to promote immune system health, digestion, and aid in the occasional problems we encounter with elimination.

Until the Vitamin Code Raw Food-Created Nutrients burst on to the scene, Fermented or Cultured Vitamins and Minerals were the most innovative forms of whole food supplementation. They still offer all their highly touted benefits. However, they do not have all of the innovation found in Raw Food-Created Nutrients.

THE VITAMIN CODE™

RAW FOOD-CREATED NUTRIENTS

When Andy Szalay cracked the Vitamin Code and began producing Raw Food-Created Nutrients that could be used to make multivitamins, there was a paradigm shift in nutritional supplements available on the market today. While Raw Food-Created Nutrients, when renatured from isolated vitamins and minerals, are not equal to the benefits of ingesting actual raw, organic, whole foods, they are as close to real food as supplementation can get.

Here's an explanation why. The next time you plant a tomato bush, pick an orange from a tree, or drive by a farm that grows peppers, you will find the inspiration for the Vitamin Code. The tomato bush, the orange tree, and that field of peppers all share a common biological trait. They absorb inorganic material from the soil and turn them into vitamins and minerals bound to the proteins, complex carbohydrates, flavonoids, glycoproteins, fibers, and other parts of the plant.

The process is simply described, and you may remember it from high school biology. The soil that these plants are grown in is replete with inorganic materials, which are known by chemists as inorganic salts. When the plants take root, they pull these inorganic salts from the ground. When sunlight is added to the process, the plant uses these inorganic salts to make vitamins and plant bound minerals. Additionally, there are other co-factors created in the growing process such as enzymes and phytonutrients. Taken together, the vitamins, minerals, and co-factors are what give the food its nutritional power in the body.

The process used to grow the vitamins and minerals for the Garden of Life Vitamin Code multivitamins mimics the process found in the plant kingdom. Each individual vitamin and mineral found in the six Vitamin Code formulations is individually grown in single batches. For the purposes of explaining the process we will focus on one mineral, selenium.

The process for growing selenium starts with a single-cell organism, in this case *Saccharomyces cerevisiae*, or baker's yeast, which we most commonly associate with bread and baked goods. *Saccharomyces cerevisiae* was chosen because it retains the complex cell structure of a plant, but it's also easy to grow. The *Saccharomyces cerevisiae* is mixed with water that has been subjected to a multi-stage purification process to ensure that it's free of any unwanted ingredients that will affect the growing process. Molasses is then added as food for the yeast, and the yeast is allowed to begin the budding and growing process.

At the same time the yeast is growing, in a separate cultivation tank the elemental or pure selenium has a specific peptide complex added to it. A peptide is a chain of amino acids that play an important role in the absorption of selenium by the yeast during the growing and metabolization process.

At the proper time in the growing process, the peptide-complex selenium is added to the growing *Saccharomyces cerevisiae*. The peptide allows the selenium to pass through the cell wall of the *Saccharomyces cerevisiae*. Without the peptide, the selenium could not penetrate the cell wall of the yeast and would remain an inorganic salt, a lifeless material. The presence of the peptide, however, allows the selenium access to the *Saccharomyces cerevisiae,* where it displaces sulfur and then imbeds itself to specific amino acids in the natural backbone protein of *Saccharomyces cerevisiae*. The result: selenium becomes part of the *Saccharomyces cerevisiae*.

In order to halt the growing process of the *Saccharomyces cerevisiae* and make the nutrients created more available, enzymes called papain (from papaya) are then added to break down the cell wall of the *Saccharomyces cerevisiae*. Once this is accomplished, the enzymes are deactivated. The enzymes chosen for this task are done so because they are susceptible to lower temperature thresholds.

The mixture is brought to 113 degrees, deactivating just the papain enzymes. More importantly, this low temperature allows other important enzymes created during the growing process inherent to *Saccharomyces cerevisiae* to live on. It is incredibly important to remember that these "Code Factors" are not *added* to the process, they are *created* by the budding and growth process. Like a plant growing in a farmer's field, the process used to grow our vitamins and minerals creates powerful Code Factors. Great lengths are taken to ensure that these Code Factors are not destroyed during the growing or cultivation process.

In addition to the growing of vitamins and minerals in *Saccharomyces cerevisiae*, the Vitamin Code also uses vitamins and minerals grown in *Lactobacillus bulgaricus*, an important probiotic. The process is very similar to the process used with *Saccharomyces cerevisiae*, with one distinct difference—the peptides used for *Lactobacillus bulgaricus* are distinct from *Saccharomyces cerevisiae* in order to assure the nutrients are effectively absorbed into the probiotic.

You may ask why the Vitamin Code uses the two different probiotic-growing processes (*Saccharomyces cerevisiae* and *Lactobacillus bulgaricus*). The answer is pretty simple. Each process contributes its own unique set of Code Factors to the final raw ingredient. By including vitamins and minerals grown in each process, you're offered a wider array of beneficial code factors not found in any other vitamin and mineral formulation available today.

GOING RAW ALL THE WAY

All this talk about the Raw Food-Created Nutrients is a great place to introduce one of the world's leading experts in raw foods as well as an author of a half-dozen books—Paul Nison. He contends that raw is the healthiest way we can eat our foods, and that raw fruits, vegetables, nuts, and seeds contain all the nutrients and enzymes that we would ever need.

Paul's journey toward eating raw started when he was twenty years old and found his health was compromised with severe digestive troubles. Paul was living in New York City, rushing through a frenzied life as a Wall Street trader, but his poor health caused him to rethink where he was headed. He discovered that eating seemed to make him feel worse. *Wait a minute*, he thought. *If what I eat is causing my troubles* . . . .

So Paul started experimenting by eliminating foods that made him feel ill. Gone were the cheeseburger and fries, the "gut-bomb" burritos, and the spicy nachos. As he simplified his diet, he discovered that the only foods that left him feeling good—even vibrant and healthy—were fresh organic fruits and vegetables, as well as nuts and seeds. But they had to be served raw.

"I finally realized that health doesn't start with what we add to our diet but with what we leave out," he said.

Paul also did some subtraction to his lifestyle. He ditched the Wall Street financial industry and resettled in West Palm Beach, where he wrote his first book in 2000 entitled *The Raw Life: Becoming Natural in an Unnatural World*, which explained how to incorporate raw foods into a cooked diet and—should the spirit lead you—how to transition to a 100-percent raw diet. These days, Paul follows a raw vegan diet, meaning he eats no processed or cooked foods or any food that comes from animals, like meat or dairy products.

Paul says that eating foods heated above 118 degrees Fahrenheit starts to deplete the enzyme potential, draining energy that the body counts on to maintain tissues and organ systems.

That's because when food is cooked above that 118 degree-and-up threshold for three minutes or longer, vitamins are destroyed, protein becomes denatured, sugar becomes caramelized, and natural fibers are broken down.

When Jordan Rubin told Paul about the exciting work being done to develop Vitamin Code multivitamins produced with raw food-created nutrients, his bushy eyebrows registered great interest. "I got excited when Jordan explained to me the whole technology behind the Vitamin Code. I'm definitely looking forward to telling the world about these powerful products because not only are they the only raw vitamins and minerals I know of, but I also believe them to be of the highest quality. It's just taking what's out there now to the next level," he said.

"There are a whole bunch of people like myself who want to take vitamins that aren't missing enzymes because they've been processed by heat," he said. "The fact that Vitamin Code multivitamins are vegan is a real plus for me, and I know people are looking for vegan raw food vitamins."

If you ask Paul why the raw food movement seems to be exploding these days, he'll cite two reasons: the desire to lose weight and the megaphone of Hollywood celebrities. Regarding the former, overweight individuals have discovered that switching to a raw food diet is an instant way to cut calorie consumption tremendously—and shed pounds that stay off. According to the Mayo Clinic, you consume only sixty calories when you eat one of these foods as a snack:

- **One Small Apple**
- **One-Half Cup of Grapes**
- **Two Plums**
- **Two Tablespoons of Raisins**
- **One and One-Half Cups of Strawberries**
- **Two Cups of Shredded Lettuces**
- **One-Half Cup of Diced Tomatoes**
- **Two Cups of Spinach**
- **Three-Fourths Cup of Green Beans**

On the other hand, a medium-sized mocha ice cream treat with candy toppings and hot fudge, topped with pistachio nuts comes out to a whopping 1,150 calories, or *twice* the amount of calories contained in *all* the fruits and vegetables just listed!

Then there are the Hollywood A-listers who've been vocal about their embracement of the raw lifestyle. Carol Alt, Danny Glover, Woody Allen, Alicia Silverstone, Demi Moore, Pierce Brosnan, Woody

Harrelson, and Angela Bassett have, at one time or another, declared their allegiance to raw foods, and some have hired personal chefs to prepare raw dishes.

Yes, a lot of folks are jumping on the raw bandwagon, but don't let that stop you from checking out a healthy way to eat that helps you lose weight and support the immune system, which can help protect you from the ravages of free radicals.

Taking Vitamin Code multivitamins, created from uncooked and unadulterated sources, not only meet the raw standard, but they will lift your life to heights you never imagined.

He Said It

"I knew it was only a matter of time before somebody with the experience in the supplement industry like Jordan Rubin would come along and figure out how to make a top-quality line of multivitamins made from raw nutrients.**"**

—Paul Nison, author and speaker about the raw lifestyle

For more information, go to www.PaulNison.com or check out Paul's newest book, The Formula for Health.

Looking to Get More Raw In Your Life?

Raw isn't eating just apples and oranges for breakfast and lunch with a tossed salad for dinner. A food processor can be used for producing taco "meat" from a mixture of soaked walnuts, cilantro, wheat-free tamari soy sauce, and cumin and coriander powder. A raw version of Shiitake chow mein begins with Shiitake mushrooms. Tahini is made from sesame seed kernels, and sunflower seeds can be blended into a pâté.

At the Vitamin Code website at **www.TheVitaminCode.com**, you'll find some exciting raw food recipes that will fit your needs whether you are looking to go totally raw or just include more raw foods into your diet. There really is no right or wrong when it comes to raw, which is another reason why so many people are embracing the lifestyle.

No matter what source you use, many recipes for raw foods entail using a dehydrator, which is a small home appliance for drying fresh food. They come in a variety of sizes and work by gently heating the air not above 118 degrees while blowing throughout the food-drying area. Dehydrators generally cost a couple of hundred dollars and up and are worth the investment if you start eating more raw foods.

THE IMPORTANCE OF ENZYMES

There's an aspect to Raw Food-Created Nutrients that we should discuss, and it's called the food enzyme theory. First, some background:

Back in the 1930s, when biochemists were discovering the last batch of vitamins and minerals like vitamin K and vitamin B6, researchers were also learning that proteins act as catalysts for all chemical reactions in the body. They called these proteins *enzymes*. Scientists initially identified eighty enzymes eighty years ago; today more than 5,000 enzymes have been discovered. Our minds can barely comprehend how complex the role of enzymes are when you consider that a single human liver cell contains at least 1,000 different enzyme systems.

Enzymes not only initiate chemical processes in the body by removing parts, adding parts, or just snipping off a piece to change their makeup, they do so quickly and efficiently. Without enzymes, life would slow to a standstill because chemical reactions inside our bodies wouldn't happen fast enough unless enzymes were part of the mix. Enzymes seem to be particularly important for proper digestion, followed by tissue and organ repair.

Enzymes do their work by reducing the energy required for the individual reactions to take place. In other words, enzymes make it easier for two proteins to react together, which is an incredible circumstance when you consider that hundreds of thousands of reactions take place in the body every minute. For example, your central nervous system is busy processing information while your digestive system is processing your last meal. Your immune system is handling the many germs and particles that have entered your body, your heart is beating, and life-giving cells are being made and replaced as other internal systems carry out a multitude of other intricate processes. All of these functions involve thousands of different enzymes.

The late Edward Howell, M.D., and author of the seminal book *Enzyme Nutrition*, was among the pioneers who began studying the role of enzymes in the late 1920s and early 1930s. After extensive clinical and laboratory research, he began sounding the alarm about the importance of eating the right foods to ensure a proper level of enzyme activity within the human body. He was particularly attentive to the role that digestive enzymes play in keeping us healthy because when the digestive tract goes off the rails, life can be miserable. Just ask anyone suffering from food poisoning or diarrhea resulting from the intestinal flora imbalance caused by taking antibiotics.

Digestive enzymes break down food so that our bodies can use the nutrients contained within that food. When food is swallowed, it moves to the stomach and then to the small intestine, followed by the large intestine. At each step along the way, specific enzymes break down different types of food. For example, an enzyme designed to digest protein has no effect on starch, and an enzyme active in the mouth may not be active in the stomach. Ideally, though, these enzymes work together, digesting food and delivering nutrients to cells to maintain their health.

To make sure that our bodies have the digestive enzymes needed to break down the proteins, starches, and fats in the foods we eat, Dr. Howell declared that it's very important to eat certain raw and fermented foods high in enzyme content. The enzymes in raw food help jump-start the process of digestion and reduce the body's need to produce digestive enzymes, he believed.

Raw foods are best since some enzymes are deactivated—a nicer word than *destroyed*—at a wet-heat temperature as low as 118 degrees Fahrenheit and a dry-heat temperature as low as 150 degrees.

It could be a design of nature that foods and liquids at 117 degrees can be touched without burning yourself, but liquids over 118 degrees will burn you. Thus, there is a built-in mechanism for determining whether or not the food we are eating still contains its enzyme content, according to Sally Fallon, author of the book, *Nourishing Traditions*.

Cooking food destroys important enzymes, said Dr. Howell, and a diet composed exclusively of cooked food puts a severe strain on the body, drawing down its reserves. If the body is constantly overstimulated to produce enzymes that *ought* to be in foods, the result over time will be inhibited functions of the body and/or nutrient deficiencies. Humans eating an enzyme-poor diet, comprised primarily of cooked food, use up a tremendous amount of their enzyme potential in the outpouring of secretions from the pancreas and other digestive organs.

The result, according to Dr. Howell, is a shortened life span, illness, and lowered resistance to stress of all types. He pointed out in his book *Enzymes for Health and Longevity* that humans and animals on a diet comprised largely of cooked food, particularly grains, have poorer health that is evident when certain organs are examined postmortem.

"Dr. Howell formulated the following Enzyme Nutrition Axiom: The length of life is inversely proportional to the rate of exhaustion of the enzyme potential of an organism. In other words, the increased use of food enzymes promotes a decreased rate of exhaustion of the enzyme potential. Another sage rule can be expressed as follows: "Whole foods give good health; enzyme-rich foods provide limitless energy," wrote Sally Fallon in *Nourishing Traditions*. Unfortunately, our diets do not consist of these health-giving foods, and even if they did, the grains, fruits, and vegetables coming from our soil-depleted field don't hold a candle to the nutritious bounty found in harvested crops prior to World War II.

While we could all stand to include plenty of raw foods in our diets—bountiful salads teeming with greens, tomatoes, and onions instead of cooked broccoli, baby carrots instead of crinkle-cut potato chips and sour cream dip, and a bowl of in-season strawberries and blueberries instead of a heaping helping of vanilla ice cream —the reality is that few people think "raw" when planning their menus. This is where supplements made from raw ingredients—such as Vitamin Code Raw Food-Created Nutrients —supplement the body with enzymes missing from cooked foods.

Enzymes are delicate dynamos. Delicate because many enzymes start to be destroyed when they reach a temperature of 118 degrees Fahrenheit, and they are obliterated when they stay at that temperature for even a miniscule period of time, which eliminates most steamed and cooked vegetables. Dynamos because these powerful biochemical catalysts are necessary for digestion, breathing, talking, moving, cellular energy, tissue and organ repair, neutralization of toxins, and brain activity. Dr. Howell said that although the body can manufacture enzymes, the more you use up your enzyme "potential"—meaning a regular diet of cooked, canned, or processed foods—the more you place yourself at risk for developing nutrient deficiencies that translate into serious health woes further down the line.

BRINGING THE MESSAGE HOME

Taking supplements with Raw Food-Created Nutrients, such as Garden of Life Vitamin Code multivitamins, keeps your body stocked with enzymes as well as living probiotics. The Vitamin Code multivitamins have been produced using Raw Food-Created Nutrients that have been uncooked, untreated, unadulterated, and untouched. In other words, these are 100 percent active and raw vitamin and mineral supplements.

The term "raw" may carry a negative connotation for you, and understandably so. Many of us don't like our meat or fish served raw, except for steak tartare aficionados and sushi fans. Or maybe you equate "raw" with those wrestling matches you see on cable featuring bouts that are "uncut, uncensored, and uncooked."

If that's the case with you, put those images aside because uncooked, enzyme-rich, untreated, and unprocessed Vitamin Code supplements can bring vitality without placing as big of a burden on the body's digestive system. I (Massoud) worked with the Garden of Life team for nearly a year to create their new line of multivitamins made with Raw Food-Created Nutrients. They are:

- **Vitamin Code Family Formula**
- **Vitamin Code Men's Formula**
- **Vitamin Code 50 & Wiser Men's Formula**
- **Vitamin Code Women's Formula**
- **Vitamin Code 50 & Wiser Women's Formula**
- **Vitamin Code Perfect Weight Formula**

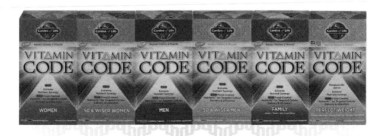

I can assure you that Grow Company and Garden of Life looked at every single ingredient in the manufacturing process and put these formulations through intensive scrutiny to make sure that every aspect of the production process remained raw so that these ingredients will be of the highest quality.

You, the individual, are the beneficiary. What Andy discovered was that a simple single-cell organism that we know as baker's yeast had the ability to transform inorganic substances like calcium carbonate and isolated crystalline nutrients into complex nutrients good for our bodies and in a form more closely resembling how humans were intended to receive their nutrients.

In other words, Andy Szalay was able to break the Vitamin Code, and because of his perseverance that stretched over three decades, our lives today can be lived better, healthier, and longer.

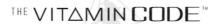
Quality Control Is Job One

by Massoud Arvanaghi

There's something else going for the Vitamin Code multivitamins besides their raw, unadulterated nature, and that's the quality control processes that we employ throughout the manufacturing process.

Let's start with the eighteen-wheel trucks delivering the raw materials—there's that *raw* word again—to our plant in Ridgefield, New Jersey. Onboard those trucks are commodities like active dry live yeast, molasses, inorganic salts, and various fruit concentrates like citrus, carrot, and alfalfa that are used in the production of Raw Food-Created Nutrients, which are used to make Garden of Life Vitamin Code multivitamins. We're talking tons of raw materials each month.

All those raw materials—which come in secured drums—are placed in a quarantined section until they can be tested by our laboratory technicians for purity. While we do accept vendor's Certificate of Analysis regarding the product's purity, we don't rely on it. That's why anything that arrives on the loading dock at our Ridgefield factory must be checked and double-checked, according to our standards, before we can start the manufacturing process. If our laboratory discovers an impurity or deviation from our specifications in the active live yeast or molasses, for example, the delivery is rejected.

Once our laboratory releases the raw materials, they are entered into the computer and can be used for production. When we make a batch of

Raw Food-Created Nutrients, we send samples of the intermediates during production back to the lab for testing throughout the manufacturing process. We're talking about a lot more than just a sample at the beginning and end; early in the process, we send a sample back to the lab every ten to thirty minutes during the production process.

Our lab runs Fourier Transfer Infrared Spectroscopy (FTIR) tests on each sample. Every individual product, intermediate, chemical, natural or synthetic ingredient has a distinct FTIR fingerprint. This fingerprint is inherent to that specific ingredient—just like the human fingerprint is inherent to the individual. The FTIR is a versatile technique that the lab chemist uses to analyze and match for the presence of specific components in a particular product.

The method gives us the ability to detect the progress of the batch at every step of production. As with most lab instruments, FTIR units are delicate pieces of equipment that are susceptible to breakdown even under the most ideal conditions, but we feel this is a worthwhile expense.

Throughout the production process, we also subject every single raw material, intermediary step, or finished product to GC analysis, GC standing for Gas Chromatography. We do this to make sure there are no residual solvents or herbicides or pesticides in our products. Although we don't claim that Raw Food-Created Nutrients are certified organic, we are certain that our product is free of additives or harmful pesticide residues. Numerous other tests are performed to make certain of the quality of the raw ingredients, intermediates, and finished products. These are testing by

Ultraviolet Spectroscopy (UV), High Performance Liquid Chromatography (HPLC), Inductively Coupled Plasma (ICP), Atomic Absorption (AA), and Karl Fischer (KF). How's that for an alphabet soup?

There are a couple of more points you should know about. The water we use in the manufacturing process is taken through several steps of purification. Even after all these purifications, a sample is sent to the lab for Total Carbon Analysis (TOC), followed by microbiological clearance before given complete go-ahead. Also, since aerobic microorganisms need fresh air to come to life and stay alive, we also "scrub" the air inside our manufacturing plant prior to bubbling it into the living microorganism.

You now have an idea of all the acronyms we use every day at the Grow Company, but we feel these tests are vital to the manufacturing process. I've condensed a lot of information here, but the day-to-day reality is that our Quality Control is exceedingly thorough—and expensive, which is why we believe that no one else in our industry even comes close to what we are doing. We're constantly upgrading our laboratory testing equipment to stay ahead and ensure that our products have the very best quality possible.

Break the Code

- The vast majority of vitamins and minerals sold in the United States are made from isolated, synthetic sources.

- Don't be fooled by bottles of vitamins that scream out "Natural" or even "Whole Food" on the packaging.

- Don't underestimate the importance of the Raw Food-Created Nutrients and live probiotics and enzymes used to create Vitamin Code multivitamins. These Raw Food-Created Nutrients are uncooked, untreated and unadulterated.

To find out more about these amazing Vitamin Code formulas, or to find a local health food retailer near you, visit us online at **www.TheVitaminCode.com.**

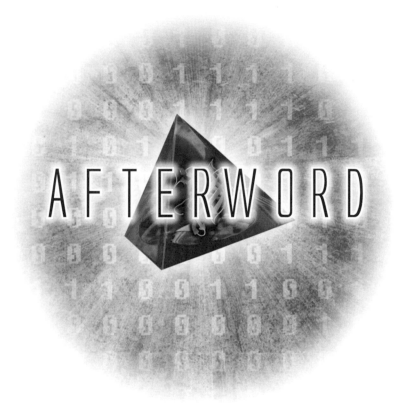

AFTERWORD

BY JORDAN RUBIN

Like you, I was spellbound by Andy Szalay's dramatic story of escaping the Iron Curtain and his subsequent scientific discoveries that cracked the Vitamin Code. Just before the release of this book, I was introduced to this remarkable gentleman for the first time, and I have to admit that I was awed. I was greatly pleased to thank him for his contributions to mankind.

When you think about it, Andy was in the right place at the right time in history, and we are the beneficiaries. He is one of those unique individuals who can observe and see things that prompt him to ask questions that no one has ever asked before. He showed us that he could examine scientific discoveries from the past and be willing to spend decades of his life expanding upon them.

Let me give you a small example how Andy thinks outside the proverbial box. In nearly all of my books, I've talked about the importance of washing your hands. It's absolutely brutal how many millions of people each day fail to wash their hands after going to the bathroom. They ignorantly leave the restroom and spread their germs on an unsuspecting public when they shake hands and interact with people. While germs may instigate disease, it is important to note that they cause the body's resistance to weaken by stressing the immune system.

Remember how I said that Andy can look at something and see a solution no one has ever thought about before? Well, when Andy was building a new Grow Company manufacturing plant in Ridgefield, New Jersey, seven years ago, he came up with a remarkably novel idea for the employee washrooms. Since he couldn't *force* males to wash up after using the urinals, he thought of a way to lead them to water, so to speak.

In Andy's restrooms, after the male completes his business at the urinal and steps away, a sensor would automatically flush the urinal. Nothing special about that: that's how millions of urinals work all over the world.

Here's where Andy's genius began. He installed a second sensor at the washbasin that would keep the restroom door locked until the faucet was turned on. In other words, someone who zipped up and tried to leave the restroom without washing his hands would find the door automatically locked. Someone who washed his hands would trip the sensor, which would automatically unlock the exit door.

Very clever.

Andy installed the system without telling his employees what he was up to. To his great pleasure and pleasant surprise, he found out that his male employees washed their hands without being told to. They walked in, used the urinal, washed their hands, and departed without incident. Germs weren't passed around the plant, and Andy viewed his experiment as a success.

Then came the day when a delivery truck driver asked to use the facilities. He planted himself in front of the urinal but skipped the hand-washing part. The door remained locked.

He pounded on the door. He made a scene. And ultimately, when someone told him how he could open the door, the truck driver was embarrassed.

Following that incident, the local fire marshal stopped by for his annual inspection, and in poking around, he discovered Andy's novel solution to hygienic cleanliness. In this OSHA-ruled world, what would happen if an unsuspecting employee was stuck inside the bathroom and a fire broke out?

So the sensor at the water faucet was removed, but at least Andy gave it a shot, which shows you a glimpse of his genius-like abilities. You would think that someone who's been responsible for some of the most significant discoveries in nutritional research in the last forty years would be well-known—even famous—among his peers. Well, I have news for you: I would say that ninety-nine out of a hundred people in the nutritional supplement industry have never heard of Andy. I hope he'll receive some well-deserved recognition following the release of this book and the Vitamin Code multivitamins from

Garden of Life, a company I started more than ten years ago.

Andy has been well-served by his successor, Massoud Arvanaghi, a brilliant researcher who has a passion for what he does. I think Massoud's the perfect person, from a creative and production side, to carry on the mantle of Andy. His loyalty and his understanding of the big picture have been instrumental in Grow Company's success. When we at Garden of Life approached Massoud and the Grow Company about producing this new category of raw food-created multivitamins, Massoud understood our passion to create the best multivitamins in the history of our industry as well as "tell the story" about Andy Szalay, the Hungarian immigrant who entered this country with the clothes on his back and a sincere hope to improve the health of others.

We began working together in the summer of 2007 to develop the Vitamin Code multivitamins, and their 2008 release is a culmination of Andy's dream, Massoud's hard work, and my vision to produce the best nutritional supplements available. We're like a three-legged stool—we all need each other.

I'm looking forward to not only sharing the story of how Andy broke the Vitamin Code, but also to carry the torch as well. Sure, the science behind the code is complicated. The easiest way to describe what Andy did—at least to me—is to stick a plant into a pot filled with soil. Next, add copious amounts of a mineral, such as chromium. Then add water and stand back. What you have two months later is a plant with high amounts of chromium—not a pot with high amounts of chromium. What Andy figured out was how to take something that was inert—chromium, for example—and insert it into the walls of a single-cell entity like *Saccharomyces cerevisiae*.

Your body is designed to recognize vitamins and minerals best when they come from food, and the healthiest and best foods for the body to recognize are eaten raw. I've been a fan of Dr. Edward Howell and his belief that eating the right foods—mainly raw and fermented enzyme-rich foods—ensure the activity of the much-needed digestive enzymes inside the body. When I learned that Andy's Vitamin Code research meant that we—I'm talking about Garden of Life here—could introduce raw food-created multivitamins, I became very excited about the possibilities. Vitamin Code multivitamins are uncooked, untreated, unadulterated, and rich in enzymes and probiotics. While they are not the same as food, they are undisturbed, user-friendly, and provided as nature intended. I believe they are as close to food as a dietary supplement can be.

In today's food world—supermarkets, restaurants, drive-thrus—very little raw food is purchased or consumed. People choose the fries over the salad. The chips over the baby carrots. Apple pie à la mode over the apple. People think they eat enough raw foods, but if I followed you into a grocery store, shopping trip after shopping trip, week after week, month after month, I would see you purchasing the same thirty-to-fifty foods over and over again. The same milk, the same cereal, the same bread, the same meat, the same TV dinners, the same soft drinks, and the same snacks, and the same boxed desserts. The amount of raw foods tossed into the shopping cart is virtually non-existent.

Each day, you and your family eat the same things over and over again, and if your diet doesn't include many raw foods, then you and the family are missing out on some of the highest-quality foods for the human body. A few of my favorite raw foods are avocados, coconuts (particularly coconut cream), mangoes, and bananas.

I'm writing this while I'm in the midst of my cross-country Perfect Weight America Tour, and when we're in a new city, the first thing I ask the locals is where to find a raw food restaurant. Then I drop by a local health food store and buy a bunch of raw snacks—fruits, nuts, seeds, and salads—and take them back to my hotel room.

While I'm not a raw food vegan, I know that heating food over 118 degrees Fahrenheit destroys or deactivates certain enzymes and changes the molecular structure of the food. Raw foods, in a nutshell (so to speak), provide nutrients the way they are found in nature: undisturbed and unadulterated.

Please know that eating raw and supplementing raw are not the same. Only eating raw can provide all the benefits, but if you don't eat raw, have a lousy diet, or have nutrient deficiencies, taking nutritional supplements containing raw food-created nutrients, like the Garden of Life Vitamin Code line, is a great way to cover those "bases" that you've been trying to cover with your old multivitamins. After crisscrossing the country during my Perfect Weight America publicity tour, I think the need is there for *all* Americans to discover the Vitamin Code.

I've been consuming Vitamin Code Raw Food-Created Nutrients since the fall of 2007, shortly after Garden of Life and Grow Company officially joined forces to produce the Vitamin Code multivitamins. There's no way I could release Vitamin Code multivitamins to the public unless I've used them, which is why I tested some early formulations.

I'm pleased with the results during a time of great stress in my life. So far in 2008, the Perfect Weight America tour has traveled more than 25,000 miles across the U.S. with a camera crew and a tour bus to promote a campaign to end obesity. Let me tell you: speaking for ninety minutes, taking questions for another thirty to sixty minutes, signing books at appearances, talking up Perfect Weight America to TV, radio, and print interviewers, and always being "on" hasn't been easy. The Saturday night red-eye flights back home to Florida have been a killer, too.

As I mentioned in the Foreword, my wife, Nicki, and I are the proud parents of three children four years of age and under. We've adopted two infants in the last year (which is a long, wonderful story in itself), and each time before I headed back out on the road on Tuesday mornings, I made a week's worth of homemade infant formula for my babies, using a list of raw ingredients that I order from all across America.

Included in this formula are vitamins and minerals in the form of Raw Food-Created Nutrients—the very same nutrients you'll find in the Vitamin Code formulas. I wouldn't trust any other vitamins and minerals to do the job.

I believe that every American who takes a multivitamin would benefit from the Raw-Food Created Nutrients contained in the Vitamin Code formulations. This is a message I want to get out, and that's the reason why I asked Massoud Arvanaghi and Mike Yorkey to write this book.

We are taking this effort very seriously, and until every American has the opportunity to "crack the Vitamin Code" by consuming Raw

THE VITAMIN CODE™

Food-Created Nutrients, our job will not be finished.

If your multivitamin doesn't have the Vitamin Code, if it doesn't contain Raw Food-Created Nutrients, then what are you paying for? I encourage you to make the Vitamin Code Raw Food-Created Nutrients a key part of your family's health and nutrition plan and enjoy the benefits of this innovative approach to supplementation.

Your Greatest Investment— Your Health

by Jordan Rubin

I hope you're ready to jump aboard the Vitamin Code bandwagon, but I would imagine there's a crucial question floating inside your head: *How much is this going to cost me?*

In today's tough economic times, that's an important consideration. With gas prices going through the roof, airline prices soaring into the stratosphere, and housing values plummeting like a rock, families and individuals have to make difficult decisions about what they spend their money on.

A 120-capsule bottle of Garden of Life Vitamin Code multivitamins—which is a month's supply and comes in different formulas for men, women, those fifty and older, and people trying to reach their perfect weight—comes at a premium price. Innovation often does. Yet Garden of Life Vitamin Code multivitamins are created using The Vitamin Code and have value that goes far beyond its cost.

Investing in your health is like investing in a long-term mutual fund. Smart investors take the time to review their options, understand the trends, and invest their money wisely to give them the best long-term return on their investment. Shouldn't we look at our long-term health in the same manner?

The main reason why Garden of Life Vitamin Code multivitamins cost more than many other multivitamins is because they are far more expensive to produce. There are more than one hundred ingredients in each Vitamin Code multivitamin formulation alone, and each tablet has twenty-three individual enzymes. Each individual vitamin and mineral is delivered to your body in the form of Raw Food-Created Nutrients. My big speech is that you get only one body, so feed it the best nutrients you can buy.

Let me remind you that the Vitamin Code multivitamins from Garden of Life not only impart the wisdom of nature, but these nutritional supplements bring the health of the past by taking advantage of the technology of today.

In other words, Garden of Life Vitamin Code multivitamins are worthy of your investment.

Raw Vitamins for Real Women

Breast Health, Bone Strength, Pregnancy, Menopause...

Life can be stressful, deciding on a multivitamin that's right for you shouldn't be. Introducing Vitamin Code™ RAW Vitamins & Minerals from Garden of Life®, the only nutritional supplements with RAW Food-Created Nutrients™, formulated with your specific health needs in mind.

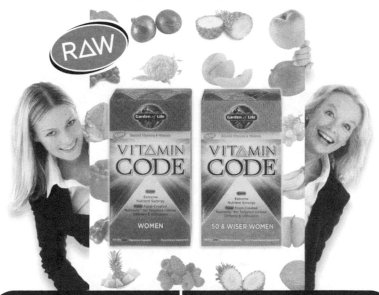

RAW

Garden of Life

VITAMIN CODE

VITAMIN CODE

WOMEN

50 & WISER WOMEN

Nature-Intended Benefits for Women†

- **Breast Health**
  Vitamin D, Vitamin E
- **Healthy Reproductive System**
  Folic Acid, Calcium, Magnesium, Zinc
- **Healthy Skin**
  Vitamin A, Vitamin C, Copper, Iron

Nature-Intended benefits for 50 & Wiser Women†

- **Bone Strength**
  Vitamins A, C, D, Calcium, Magnesium, Zinc
- **Healthy Heart & Blood Pressure††**
  Vitamin B Complex, Vitamins C & E
- **Memory and Concentration**
  Vitamin B Complex, Vitamins C, D, E

RAW • Vegan • Gluten Free • Binder Free
100% Active Ingredients • Live Enzymes & Probiotics

VITΛMIN CODE™
Beyond Vitamins & Minerals

Garden of Life®

www.RawVitamins.com

Empowering Extraordinary Health®

† These statements have not been evaluated by the Food and Drug Administration. This product is not intended to diagnose, treat, cure or prevent any disease.
†† To help maintain blood pressure levels already within the normal range.

Raw Vitamins for Real Men

Prostate Health, Energy, Good Digestion, a Healthy Heart...

Life can be stressful, deciding on a multivitamin that's right for you shouldn't be. Introducing Vitamin Code™ RAW Vitamins and Minerals from Garden of Life®, the only nutritional supplements with RAW Food-Created Nutrients™, formulated with your specific health needs in mind.

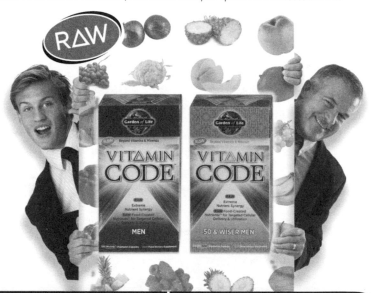

Nature-Intended Benefits for Men†

- **Mental & Physical Energy**
  Vitamin B Complex, Chromium
- **Healthy Stress Response**
  Vitamins A, C, E, Vitamin B Complex, Selenium
- **Optimal Digestion**
  Live Probiotics and Enzymes, Vitamin D

Nature-Intended benefits for 50 & Wiser Men†

- **Healthy Prostate**
  Vitamin E, Lycopene, Selenium, Zinc
- **Memory and Concentration**
  Vitamin B Complex, Vitamins C, D, E
- **Healthy Heart & Blood Pressure††**
  Vitamin B Complex, Vitamins C & E

RAW • Vegan • Gluten Free • Binder Free
100% Active Ingredients • Live Enzymes & Probiotics

VITΛMIN CODE™
Beyond Vitamins & Minerals
www.RawVitamins.com

Garden of Life®
Empowering Extraordinary Health®

Raw Vitamins for Real Families

Immune System Support, Energy, Healthy Eyes, Joint & Bone Health...

Life can be stressful, deciding on a multivitamin that's right for your family shouldn't be. Introducing Vitamin Code™ RAW Vitamins & Minerals from Garden of Life®, the only nutritional supplements with RAW Food-Created Nutrients™ formulated with your family's health needs in mind.

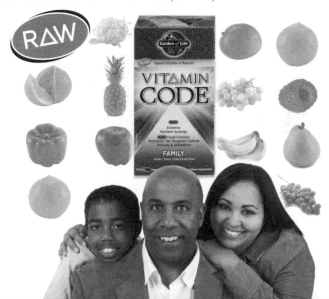

Nature-Intended Benefits for the Family†

- **Immune Support**
  Vitamins A, C, Selenium, Zinc
- **Healthy Joints & Bones**
  Vitamins A, C, D, Calcium, Magnesium, Zinc
- **Mental & Physical Energy**
  Vitamin B Complex, Chromium, Iron

- **Optimal Digestion**
  Live Probiotics and Enzymes, Vitamin D
- **Healthy Heart**
  Vitamin B Complex, Vitamins C & E
- **Eye Health**
  Vitamins A, C, E, Zinc

RAW • Vegan • Gluten Free • Binder Free
100% Active Ingredients • Live Enzymes & Probiotics

VITAMIN CODE™
Beyond Vitamins & Minerals
www.RawVitamins.com

Garden *of* Life®
Empowering Extraordinary Health®

† These statements have not been evaluated by the Food and Drug Administration. This product is not intended to diagnose, treat, cure or prevent any disease.

Raw Vitamins for Your Perfect Weight

Metabolism, Energy, Carb Cravings, Hunger...

Life can be stressful, deciding on a multivitamin that's right for your diet program shouldn't be. Introducing Vitamin Code™ RAW Vitamins & Minerals from Garden of Life®, formulated with your weight management goals in mind.

Perfect Weight AMERICA™

VITAMIN CODE™ Perfect Weight provides you:

Made with Raw Vitamins & Minerals to nourish your body as nature intended

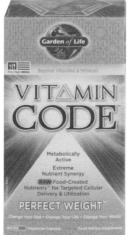

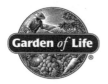
Garden of Life®

Empowering Extraordinary Health®

- **Weight Management Support**
  - Helps control stress-related weight gain[†]
  - Helps control stress-related appetite[†]
  - Helps control stress-induced overeating[†]
  - Helps reduce stress-related carb cravings[†]
- **Energy and Stress Management Support**
  - Boosts energy and reduces fatigue[†]
  - Promotes emotional well-being[†]
  - Helps increase resistance to fatigue, stress, and tension[†]
- **Overall Extraordinary Health**
  - Supports healthy cardiovascular function[†]
  - Helps support healthy blood sugar levels[†]
  - Promotes healthy inflammatory response[†]
  - Helps promote mental clarity and concentration[†]

Change Your Diet! • Change Your Life! • Change Your World!™

Vegan • Gluten Free • Binder Free
100% Active Ingredients • Live Enzymes & Probiotics

[†] These statements have not been evaluated by the Food and Drug Administration. This product is not intended to diagnose, treat, cure or prevent any disease.

www.RawVitamins.com